THE PRACTICE RECEPTIONIST

The Practice Receptionist

Book 1

MICHAEL DRURY
Professor of General Practice, University of Birmingham

RADCLIFFE MEDICAL PRESS

27 Park End Street, Oxford OX1 1HU

British Library
Cataloguing in Publication Data

Drury, M. (Michael), 1926 –
The Practice Receptionist.
Bk. 1
1. Great Britain. General practice.
Medical receptionists. Duties – Manuals
I. Title
651.3′743

ISBN 1–870905–88–1

Designed and typeset by Oxprint, Oxford

Printed and bound in Great Britain by
Alden Press, Oxford

Contents

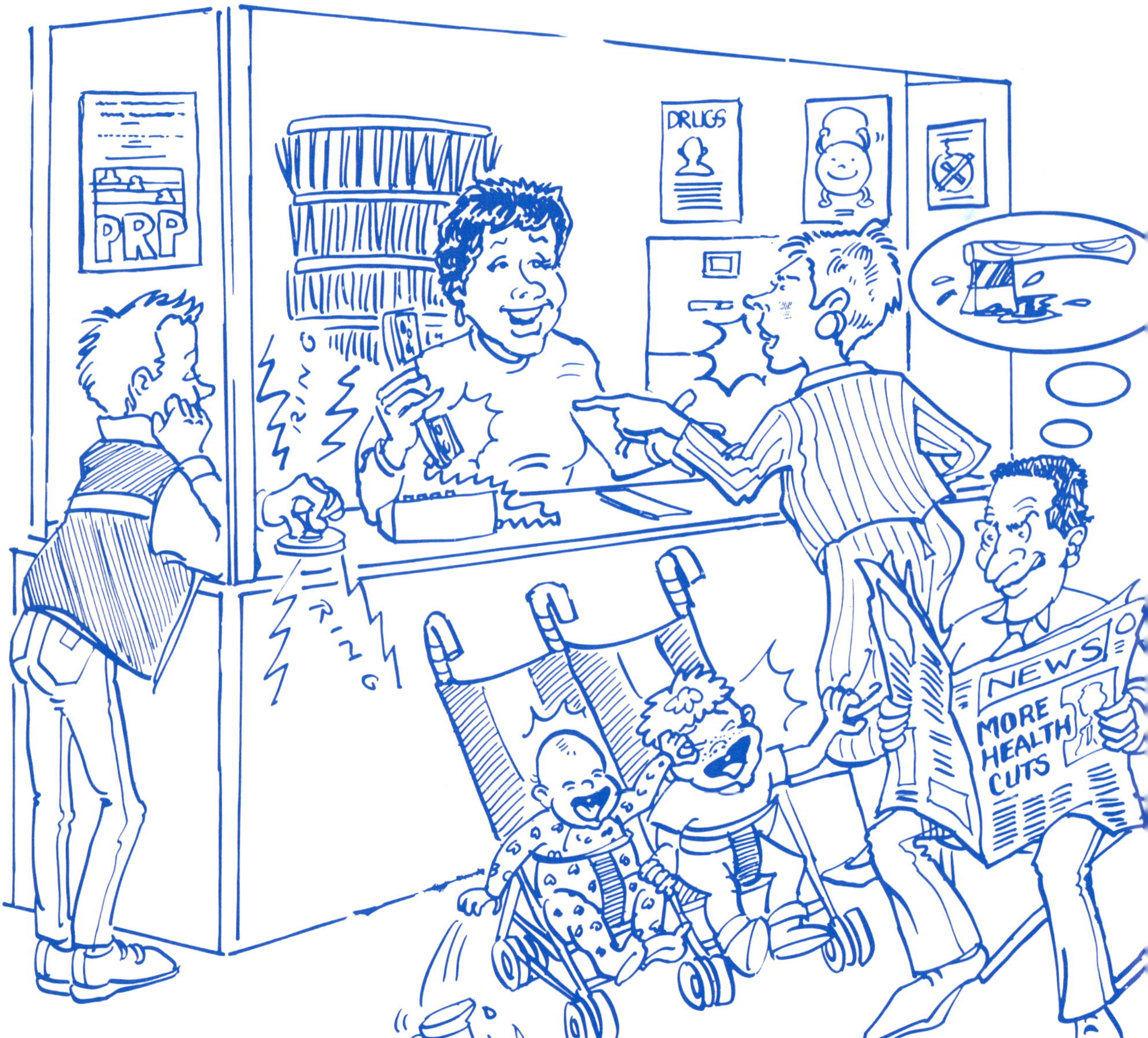
PRP
DRUGS
RING
RING
NEWS
MORE HEALTH CUTS

Preface

The first person with whom a patient makes contact in the National Health Service is most commonly the receptionist in general practice. Failings at this point may seriously affect the care of patients. This book is designed to accompany the PRACTICE RECEPTIONIST PROGRAMME which will help a receptionist improve her skills and sensitivities.

There are now over 70,000 receptionists at work in this field but despite this large number the opportunities for receptionists to meet their colleagues and to receive continuing education have, until now, been very limited. I hope that this situation will now be remedied and that this book is a contribution to a programme which will develop much further.

It is a pleasure to acknowledge the help of those who have contributed. They include a host of receptionists and practice managers with whom I have worked and some of whom attended the pilot courses. More specifically I acknowledge Lyn Shields, Merrill Whalen, Alec and Barbara Stewart, Mollie McBride, Lynne Perry and the editorial board of the Royal College of General Practitioners.

Finally, I must thank Andrew Bax who has been responsible for co-ordinating the whole project.

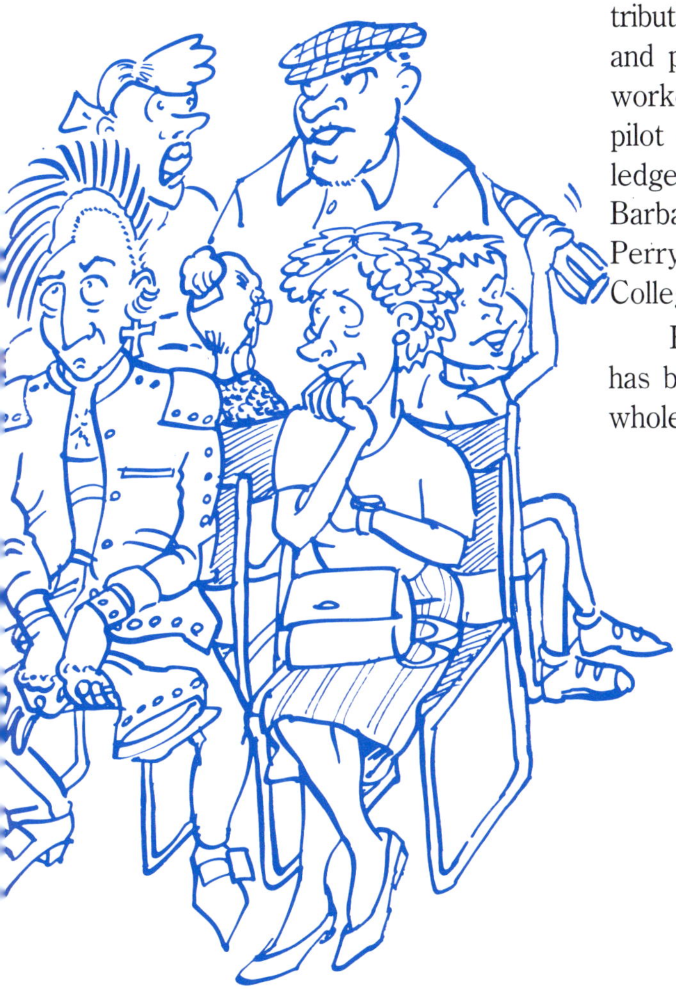

Michael Drury
January 1988

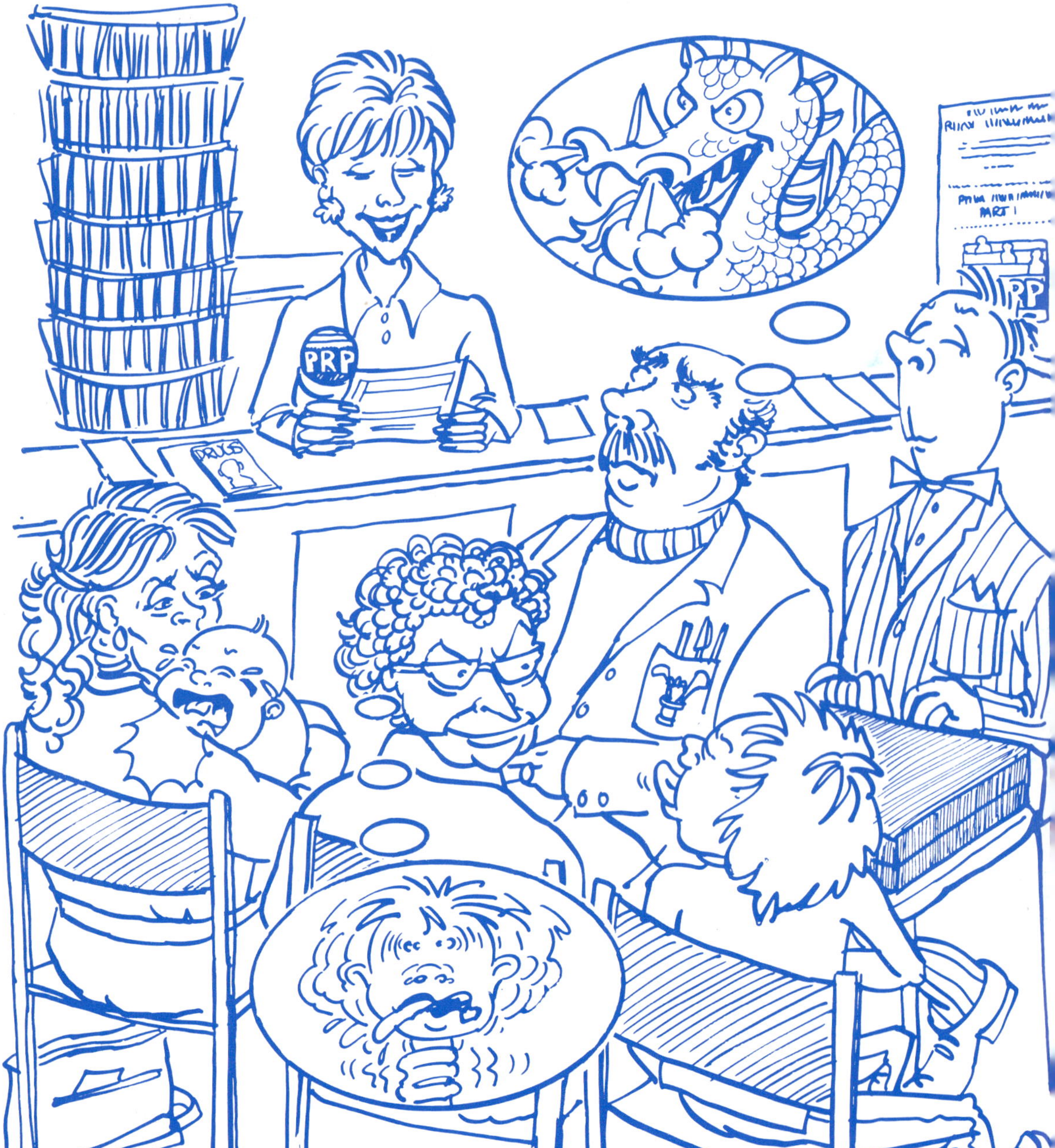

PRP
DRUGS

1

PATIENTS AND FEELINGS

The National Health Service is said to be the largest employer in Europe. Whether that is true or not it is certainly a very complex organisation. Like any large business it is quite difficult even for senior people to know where to go or whom to ask if problems arise, so how much more difficult it must be when a patient feels in trouble. Making a start is often the hardest thing to do and this is where good receptionists comes into their own, for throughout the Health Service nearly everyone starts with them. The ease with which the patient gets into the system can be absolutely critical in shaping the way the patient presents his or her problem to the doctor or the nurse, if the receptionist does not do a good job the patient may not get the help he or she needs.

When we talk about 'ease' we do not necessarily imply speed, though that may be important, we mean something more subtle than that. We mean making a patient feel comfortable, making them feel that there is nothing making life more difficult than it already is. This feeling of 'ease' becomes even more important if a patient is tired, worried, or is ill and frightened. It becomes even more important if you as a receptionist do not know that the last experience a patient had at a surgery was the feeling that everything was against him and that this is determining his behaviour.

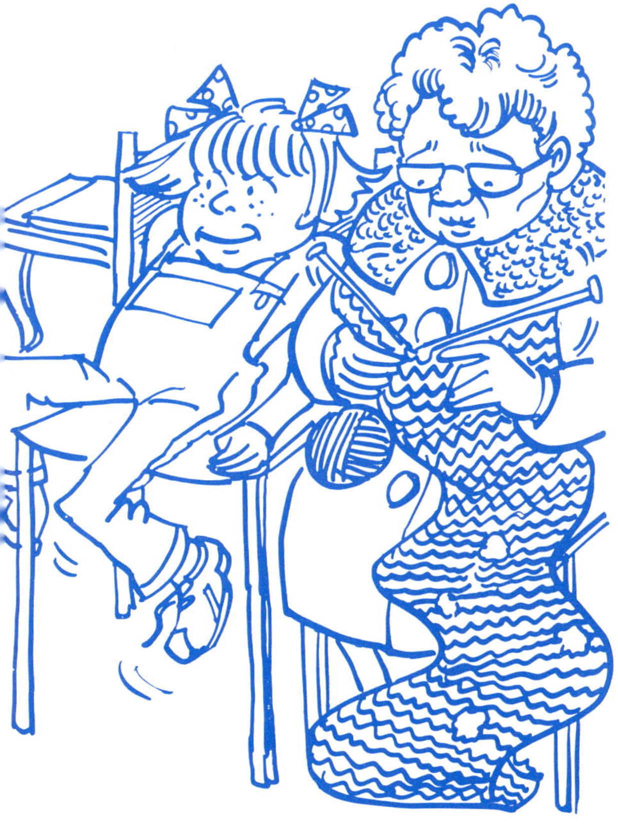

The skills required to help patients in this way are referred to as 'behavioural' skills and they can be learnt. They are affected by the attitudes we hold. For example, you may dislike teenagers. This may be due to experiences that you had earlier in life, or in a different situation, or to the opinions of other people you respect. This attitude may be deeply ingrained and may be quite difficult to eradicate, but if you know about it then it need not necessarily affect the way you behave. You may still be able to appear very welcoming to teenagers. This is acting, but there is nothing dishonest about it. We all act a lot of the time — using our tone of voice, our facial expressions and our body positions and movements to convey something more than just the words we say. Doctors in training try to improve their skills at this in a variety of different ways. One that has been recognised as being particularly useful is role play, another even more sophisticated is to use video recordings of their consultations and then to analyse them, either by themselves or with a group of colleagues. By using these techniques they can identify barriers to establishing good relationships with patients and learn how to avoid them.

Of course there is theory behind this practice and much of it is not peculiar to meetings between doctors and patients but is common to all sorts of interactions between people. In this chapter we will look at some of the factors that affect behaviour and see how they can be understood and used in practice. Some of these factors will be common to all patients and some will be peculiar to the particular patient and the particular illness.

> **?** How do you welcome people? Do you welcome all people in the same way? If not, what is it that makes you treat people differently?

ANXIETY AND FEAR

Patients are always anxious when going to visit the doctor. There are several reasons for this.

Many patients will be worried that their symptom is the first sign of serious disease. This is occasionally enough to prevent them from coming even if they can recognise the consequences of that decision. 'If I have cancer I would rather not know' is quite a common remark to overhear and the patient may even avoid talking about the lump in the breast, the cough, or the bleeding from the back passage. This is another reason why we must not put up any barriers that will stop the indecisive patient from attending.

A patient may not be so worried about the disease as about the social consequences of it. A patient may worry that the doctor will stop them working, stop them pursuing their hobby, make unpleasant restrictions on their diet and so on. All these may add to their anxiety.

The seeds of these fears may have been sown by others. Conversations with friends and 'well-wishers' may so distort the perceptions of the nature of the disease that its consequences loom out of all proportion to its severity. 'My brother had that and he had to have his leg off!' is not designed to maintain confidence in a patient suffering from repeated cramps. It is generally true that the greater the measure of uncertainty within the patient the greater the risk of influence by others and distortion by oneself.

Some people will be frightened about investigations that might be required. This feeling may range from a fear of endoscopic examinations and injections down to the simple fear of taking off their clothes and being examined. It isn't necessarily a fear of what is being done. More commonly it is a fear of how they think they will behave. Shall I faint? Shall I cry out? Shall I be unable to sit still? Finally there is the fear of seeming foolish and presenting something so trivial that they are wasting the doctor's time. Many patients, when reassured that there is nothing to worry about, say 'I am sorry to have wasted your time' when the only sensible thing they could have said was 'I am very glad it was a waste of time'.

All these worries can be exacerbated by the receptionist's behaviour. A brusque and unsympathetic manner across the desk or over the telephone; a reception area that is the scene of frenetic activity instead of ordered calm; austere premises or an unwelcoming and impersonal method of calling patients will all make matters worse and can, with care, be avoided.

? Have your experienced the kind of feelings of fear described in this section?

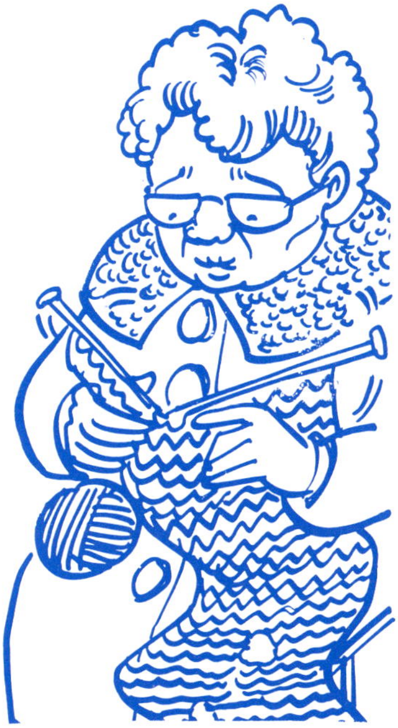

? How do you react when you are afraid?
How would you like your fear to be treated?

PERSONAL CHARACTERISTICS

We have to recognise that the patient is a unique personality with individual characteristics dependent on a very complex interaction of components.

These are partly genetic and partly a sum of life's experiences. Together they will determine how the patient reacts to his illness, to the practice, and to the individual doctor.

The patient will belong to a certain group in the community and will have the expectations, values, and attitudes of that group. These expectations will be very different for a new mother or, say, a middle-aged school teacher, or from yours — the receptionist's. The patient will be someone's son or daughter, someone's brother or spouse, and will come from a group which may be a religious or racial minority within society. Their social standing may be that of a poor or a wealthy person, that of an employer or an employee, and all these factors create expectations which will be directed at the receptionist, the practice and the doctor.

The personality of the patient will have developed in the very early years of life, we shall consider some personality types later in this chapter. Much of this personality will depend upon experiences with parents or those who cared for the patient in the early stages of life, these experiences will shape his innermost feelings and the way he reacts to the outside world. Some people feel they have to battle more with others and some are better able to cope with difficult situations.

In the doctor's surgery, as we have seen, the effect of illness is clearly one of the most important influences upon the patient's behaviour. Their attitude to that illness will be determined by their age, their personality, their social characteristics, and all their previous experiences. Reaction to the stress of any illness depends upon the resilience that the patient posesses and will vary enormously. We all have friends or colleagues who demonstrate this, some being apparently able to endure pain stoically and others succumbing immediately. We may believe we can recognise where we come upon this scale and may wish it were different or even feel guilty about it. Some people seem to have a greater capacity than others for converting mental anguish, such as troubled personal relationships, into physical symptoms, such as headache, diarrhoea, giddiness or fatigue.

Some of this behaviour is conditioned by our previous experiences with illness, doctors or hospitals, and the earlier in life that experience came the more profound is likely to be its effect. For example, a person may have been told that something 'wouldn't hurt' and when it did they may not trust doctors in future. For this reason doctors are now more honest, especially with children. In later life patients are more likely to be affected by behaviour that seems to indicate that the doctor does not care, or that he ignores people as individuals. This may make people very reluctant to present symptoms, a reluctance which could be disasterous in the case of early symptoms of serious disease. Conversely, a patient who has received kind and effective treatment will seek help more readily and at an appropriate time. We all feel we have to bang continuously on the door we believe to be locked but not if it opens readily at a touch.

The influence of some personal characteristics

As a receptionist it will be apparent to you that a variety of patterns of human behaviour parade through the waiting area. In the situation in which you work they are almost all coloured and shaped by illness and the defence mechanisms that people have developed in order to help them to cope. As we have seen the factors shaping this behaviour are incredibly complex, so the results are likely to be very varied, but it is possible to recognise the features of certain personalities which commonly present. Recognition helps us all as professionals to deal with them better.

Dependence

Everyone begins life by being dependent. As an infant we are totally dependent and gradually we begin to achieve a balance between our needs for independence and our needs for being cared for or being loved. When we become ill or feel that we are ill our need to be dependent increases and we need a bit of 't.l.c.' (tender loving care). In some people this need for dependency is highly developed, they feel their needs are urgent or pressing, so delay will make them particularly anxious and irritable. This sort of patient finds any problem regarding health too difficult to cope with and believes that unless they direct their anger and disappointment at those trying to help they may be ignored. People like this tend to frustrate and anger the professionals who are dealing with them and this compounds the difficulties.

Excessive independence

Another group of people seem to want to demonstrate to everyone that they can cope. They are either the strong, silent types or extroverts who will reject advice, rarely complain, resent attending the surgery, regard health education and preventive medicine with scorn and set up a variety of vibrations and emotions in receptionists and doctors. They also have a tendency to have problems with their personal relationships. They are anxious to conceal emotions such as fear, love, or anger, which might imply dependency, and they are reluctant to admit when trouble comes that any part of the fault could lie with them. Their excessive independence becomes a hazard to their social or physical well-being and has to be considered by the carer.

Anger

When a patient demonstrates hostility it may or may not be you who are the target. Some people have developed a pattern of responding to any sort of problem by being suspicious and picking a quarrel. They feel that they live in a hostile environment and that people and events conspire against them. They will tend to blame others for their illness and may accuse the doctor and staff of a variety of errors, discourtesy, neglect or indifference. People like this may try to provoke others into a hostile response to them so that they can show that their own anger is justified. It requires a considerable measure of control to avoid being provoked, yet on the other hand it is equally damaging to ignore complaints, as this will exacerbate the problem. It is best to deal with anger by agreeing how troublesome such things must appear to such a sensitive person, who is trying to cope with an illness as well. This sort of agreement will usually allow the patient and the receptionist to co-operate with each other on an agreed plan.

> ? In your experience, what are the most effective methods of demonstrating your understanding of a patient's emotions?

> ? Ask yourself if you have ever been angry with the 'wrong' person, in a shop perhaps? How do you deal with anger in the patient?

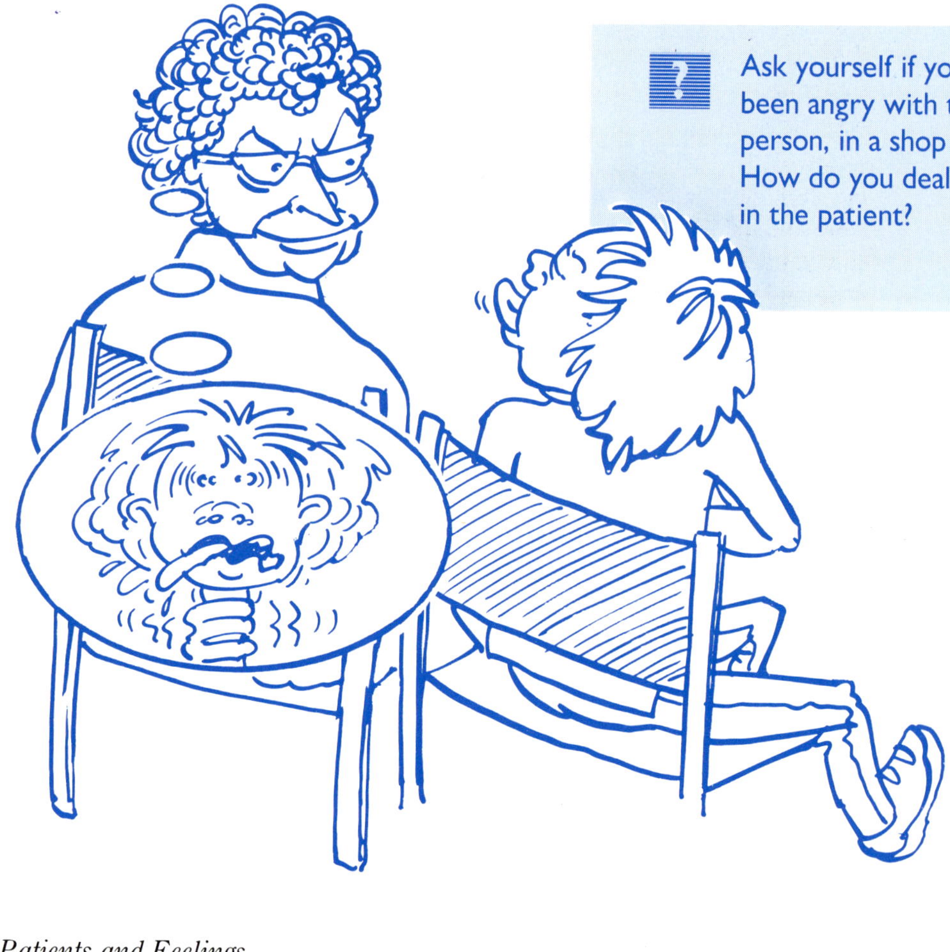

Superiority

Self-esteem is a vital component of personality. We need to feel worthwhile and to believe that we have attained some of the standards that we have set ourselves. Most of us have a balance that leaves us thinking that we have not done too badly even if we could do better. There are some people whose early development has left them with a need to demonstrate constantly that they are superior, in appearance, social position, intelligence, or in physical strength. They are almost certain to appear arrogant and demanding and will look for weakness in the receptionist or the doctor so that these can be exploited. One common feature of such behaviour is that they will always seek the attention of the most senior person; the practice manager rather than the receptionist, the senior partner rather than the trainee. They are clearly 'Very Important People' and must be treated as such. They have a great capacity for irritating staff who are made to feel they cannot be trusted.

Retreat

Most people who are ill retreat from the world to a greater or lesser degree. To a certain extent this is important and beneficial since it allows the patient rest and refuge from the troubles of the world. Sometimes the degree of retreat can be such that the real world disappears and a fantasy world appears in its place. Normal relationships with other people tend to be avoided and they shun close friendships. This leads them to appear rude and indifferent to others when in fact they are lonely and vulnerable. It is yet another reason why patients arriving at the reception desk may be rude and unco-operative.

There are many other 'types' of personality that could be described, although there is a danger of placing people in neat boxes when the variations and combinations are so great. Some people have depressive symptoms and are flat and withdrawn. Others achieve this state, without a depressive illness, by being excessively controlled. In both cases no emotion is allowed to manifest itself. Yet others may be dominated by self pity or make excessive demands upon a doctor, perhaps because of fantasies of falling in love with him or her. All of these can affect the pattern of behaviour of patients and an understanding of the nature of behavioural problems can help a receptionist in her work. We must not forget that doctors and receptionists also will be included in these behavioural groups!

> ? When a patient is angry and difficult, how do you react? Do you find it difficult to be sympathetic?

WHAT CAN WE DO ABOUT IT?

It can be understood from all we know about patients' fears that the dice are loaded against them. They have anxieties about their health and behaviour. They are in a strange place, sometimes feeling very alone, and are fearful of the outcome. If they then enter an apparently hostile environment at the reception desk it is a wonder they do not turn and run — and occasionally they do!

As the role of the receptionist is to create a bridge, not a barrier, between the doctor and the patient, it is important to identify features that influence the interaction between the two.

Welcoming the patient

The first encounter between the patient and the receptionist is of critical importance. In this section we will only consider encounters 'face to face' (we will deal with telephone encounters elsewhere). Communication has two important components, verbal and non-verbal, and they are both equally important. The verbal component consists of the words that are chosen and the manner in which they are used.

In a book written for medical students we invited the reader to consider this piece of dialogue:

He: Marmalade, please.
(a moment later)
He: *(louder)* Marmalade please.
She: Mmm?
He: Please will you pass the marmalade?
She: Oh the marmalade. Of course.
He: Thank you.

(Introduction to General Practice (1979) *Drury & Hull (Bailliere))*

We commented that this was not a very exciting piece of dialogue and all that could be inferred from it was that a man and a woman were having breakfast together and that she seemed somewhat distracted. If it was part of a theatrical dialogue we could ask you to consider how actors and a producer would handle it in four different situations:

1 They are honeymooners
2 The woman has just poisoned the marmalade with cyanide
3 He has just discovered her infidelity
4 She has just read in the paper that her shameful sex-life has been exposed

Under these circumstances, without changing the words, it would have been necessary for the actors to portray love, guilt, anger or fear in the tone of voice used. If we then look at the breakfast taking place, a whole range of other non-verbal factors should be considered. The clothes they are wearing, the expressions on their faces, the way they sit or stand and the gestures they make, all add to the picture. Of course in the theatre the actors are trying to convey meaning and emotion, whereas in real life, patients and receptionists may be trying to conceal or mask their feelings. Nevertheless something of them will always show, even if it is only an indication that concealment is taking place. Using this knowledge the receptionist will try to appear welcoming and receptive. The tools that you have for this include your appearance, your facial expression, your stance, the words you use and the way that you use them. They will also include the speed with which you act.

If you have a chance to do role play or to watch performances on video these are all things that you should look out for and see how they can be developed and improved.

Another factor we need to consider at this point is the information which has to be communicated. The words we use may mean different things to different people. This is most apparent when we meet people whose first language is not English, but it is also a barrier between people who come from different social backgrounds and whose vocabulary or regional dialect is different. It is also very important to realise that medical words may not be understood at all. People may have quite bizarre ideas about their physiology or anatomy so it is useful to ask whether what has been said is understood. In a later chapter we shall be stressing the issue of confidentiality which is of paramount importance at the reception desk. It is is not easy to reconcile the ideas of making reception easily available, and therefore 'open', with confidentiality, which has to be 'closed'. Some practices have developed ways in which this can be done and these can be explored in your group sessions.

Waiting

It is inevitable that patients going to see the doctor have to spend some time waiting. Most people will be resigned to waiting for a period providing it is comfortable and that they know that they will receive sufficient time and consideration as a result. Waiting rooms vary enormously. Some are large and impersonal, some small and intimate, the more that a waiting room resembles a factory the more likely it is that the patient will feel no-one cares about him or his illness. The ability to tolerate waiting depends on a number of factors. It is quite closely related to age. The younger you are, the less easy it is to bear it. Some old patients actually seem to enjoy the waiting for it introduces a change in their lives and gives them some companionship but it is always best to try to keep the waiting period as short as possible.

There are other factors involved. It is much easier to wait if you feel reasonably comfortable. If it is cold or noisy, or the seats are uncomfortable, it gets more difficult, especially if you feel unwell. The anxious patient will find it much less tolerable, as will the ill patient. There are times when it is possible to have a fairly good idea of the length of time that a patient will have to wait and to make preparations for this. You know, for example, that you have to turn up at the airport an hour before the plane is due to depart so you are prepared for such a wait, as time extends beyond the anticipated period it begins to affect you more and this is made much worse if you do not know how long the delay will be. If you have little else to do that morning you may accept delay in the surgery waiting room graciously but if you have fractious children with you, or left at home, if you have another appointment elsewhere that is equally important to you, you may begin to vent your displeasure upon the receptionist. It is a common annoyance to receptionists that patients do this and yet, when greeted later by an apologetic doctor, reply that it is quite alright, they understand how busy he is! It cannot be emphasised too strongly how important this waiting period is. It will generate feelings of bitterness and irritation. It is damaging to the patients self-esteem and, even if anger is rarely directed at the doctor openly, it will handicap the consultation that eventually takes place. Thus it will diminish the doctor's ability to help the patient.

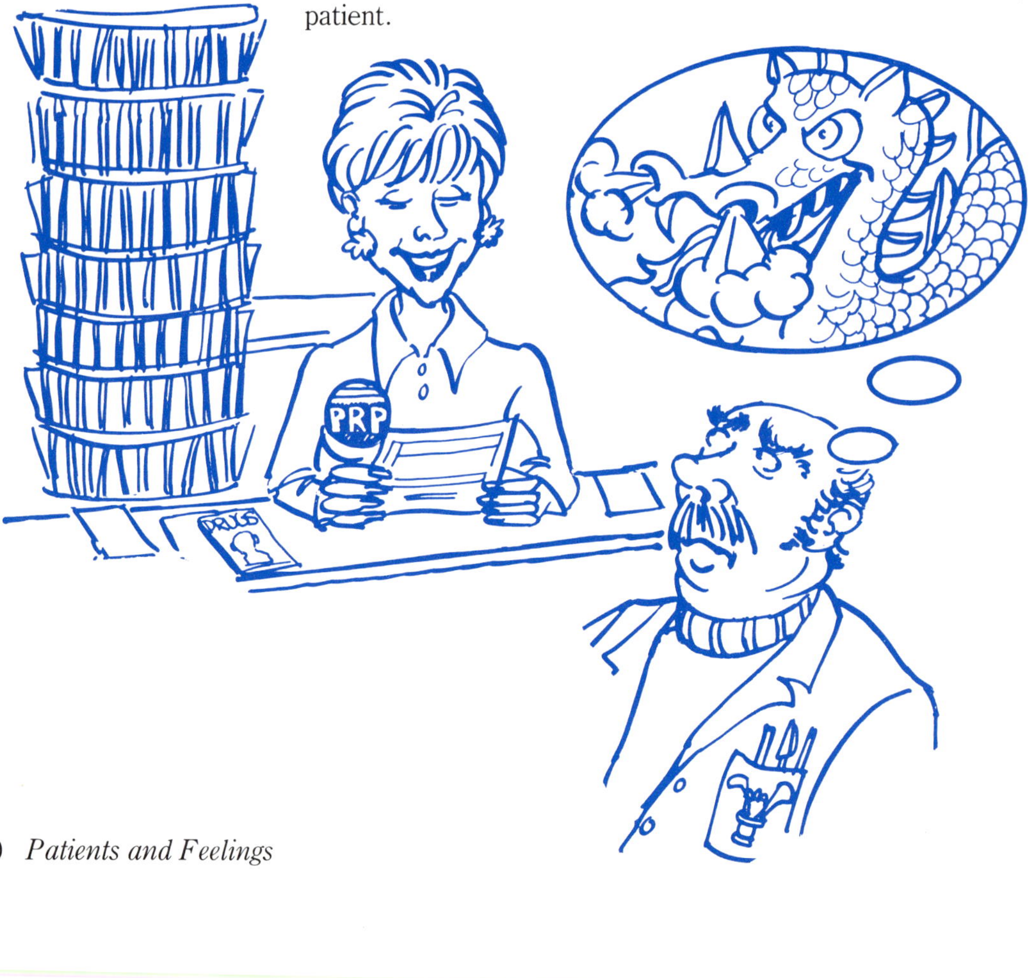

What sort of patients annoy you? Why do they, and what can you do to control this annoyance more effectively?

How can you can make waiting more tolerable for the variety of patients who attend your surgery?

How can you make your reception area and your behaviour more welcoming?

Human behaviour is infinitely variable and infinitely fascinating. There is certainly no more important part of a receptionist's work than gaining the behavioural skills that help the care of patients.

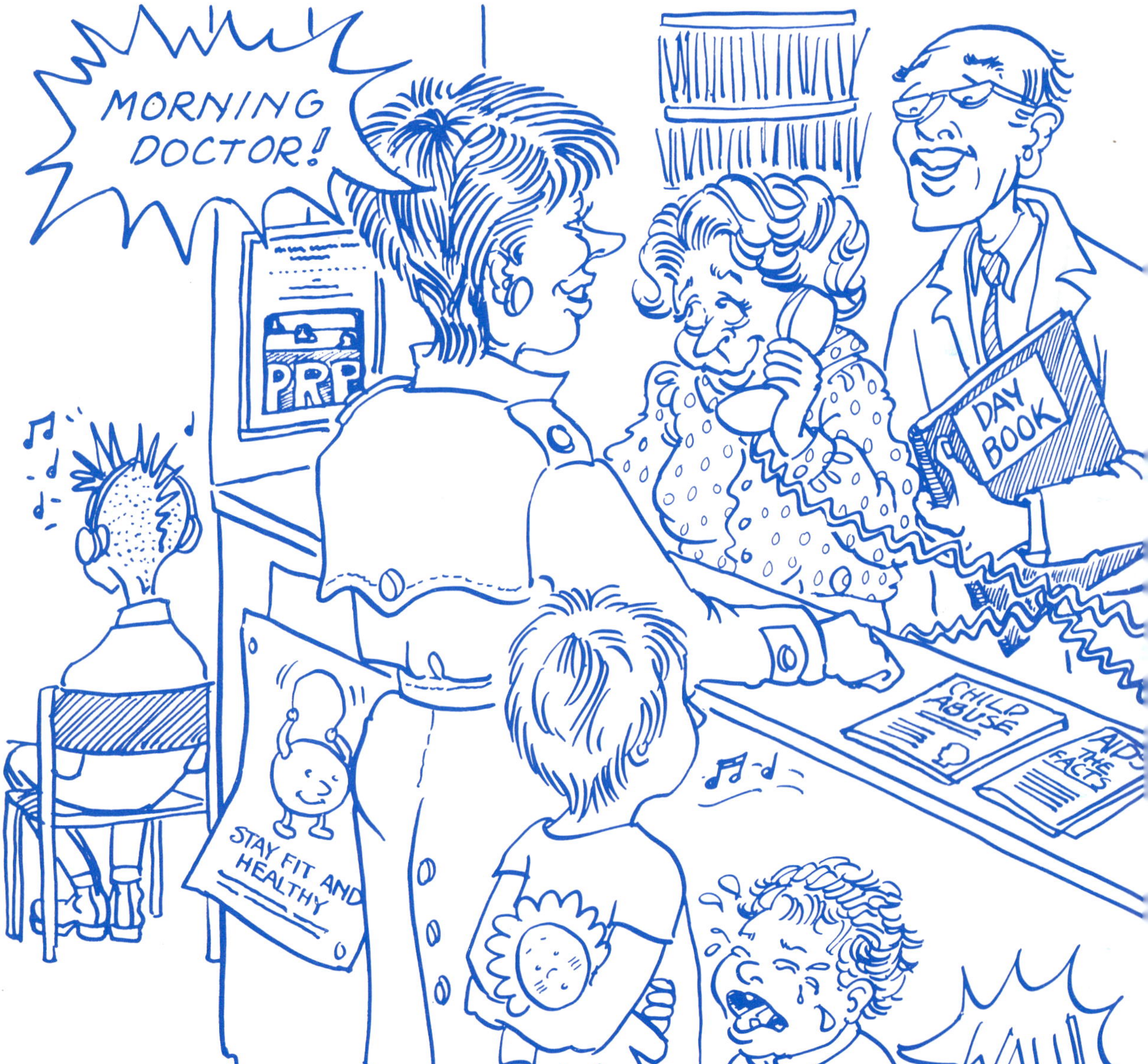
MORNING DOCTOR!
PRP
DAY BOOK
CHILD ABUSE
AIDS THE FACTS
STAY FIT AND HEALTHY
WAH!

2 COMMUNICATION

Communicating with people is far and away the most important and skilled of all the receptionist's tasks. She is the first contact the patient has with the health service in the case of almost all illnesses. She has to face a variety of situations ranging from dealing with a panicking relative faced with a life-threatening emergency to understanding a complex list of drugs needed by a patient. The ability to be calm and efficient at the same time as being warm and caring requires great skill and often creates the atmosphere that either makes or mars the subsequent consultation between the patient and a doctor or nurse.

When we try to teach someone a skill there are always two steps to be taken. This is the same whether we are learning to change a tyre or to take out an appendix. First we have to teach the theory behind the activity and demonstrate the way in which the different procedures are carried out, then we have to observe them performing the task until we are certain of competence. Learning communication skills is no different. This section of the book will cover the theory behind these activities but will be incomplete unless observations are added during some of the training sessions. This can be done using role-play or the video camera.

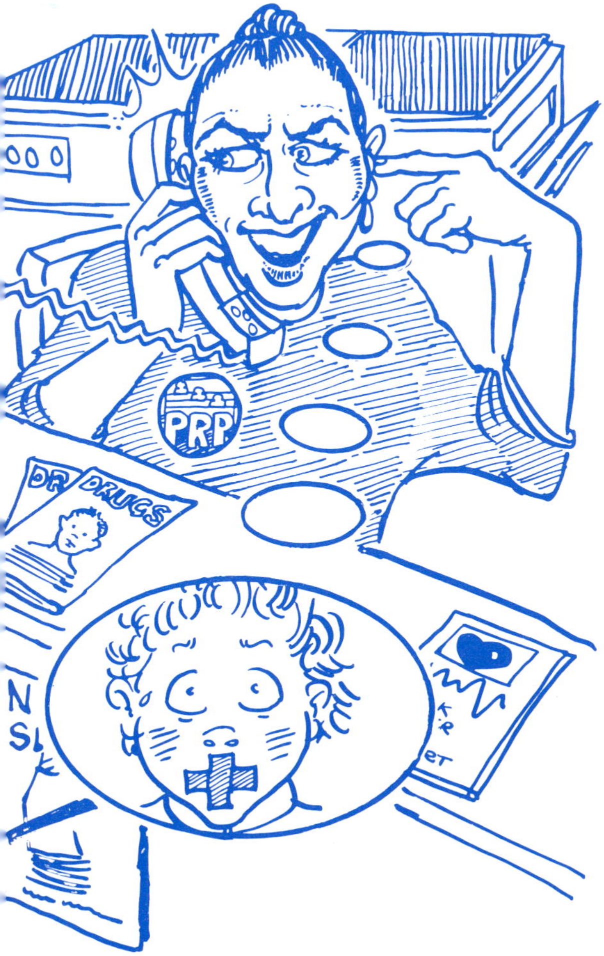

There are four ways in which a receptionist will use communication skills at work. She will have face-to-face meetings with patients (these are the key part of her work); she will talk to patients and others over the telephone; she will deal with other health care workers both on the phone and face-to-face; and finally she will have to communicate in writing.

FACE-TO-FACE MEETINGS WITH PATIENTS

These mostly take place in the reception area. Here nearly everyone who attends is anxious to some degree which, as we have already seen, affects their behaviour. The receptionist who can recognise this and cope with it is already half-way to becoming a good communicator.

At the reception desk the patient needs to

feel that he or she has the undivided attention of a person who is doing her best to make the experience as welcoming and non-threatening as possible. One way of making a patient feel at ease is to welcome him by name. Thus the receptionist who has cultivated a good eye for faces and a good memory for names is invaluable.

It is very easy for the person working at the reception area to be distracted by other happenings — the telephone may be ringing or the doctor or other colleagues may interrupt to ask for notes and so on. This is not only bad manners — you would not interrupt a conversation between two people in other circumstances — but, more importantly, it breaks the relationship between the receptionist and the patient and may prevent her from getting important information right.

Concern for the patient can be conveyed in a number of ways apart from giving undivided attention. Eye-to-eye contact and smiling are very important forms of non-verbal communication. It is surprising how some people manage to convey a sense of being unhurried and interested, even when they are under pressure, simply by making all their actions appear calm and smooth. An opening phrase such as 'Can I help you?' completes the first step of greeting the patient and lessening his anxiety.

When the patient replies to this by making their first request he is naturally hoping for a positive response. The word 'yes' has an emotional impact that shapes feelings in quite a different way from the word 'no'. It is often possible to answer a request with 'yes' even when you know that you are going to have to negotiate a different answer with the patient later. Take, for example, the patient who telephones for an appointment when you know that you are overbooked already and the doctor has to leave early, or the patient who is asking for a repeat prescription when you know that they should be seen by the doctor. There is a natural tendency to begin by saying 'no', but a compromise will be quicker, make the patient happier, and will show that you seem to be working for the same thing rather than in competition. Because of this the response 'yes', followed by the qualification 'but we are very booked up and, though we could fit you in

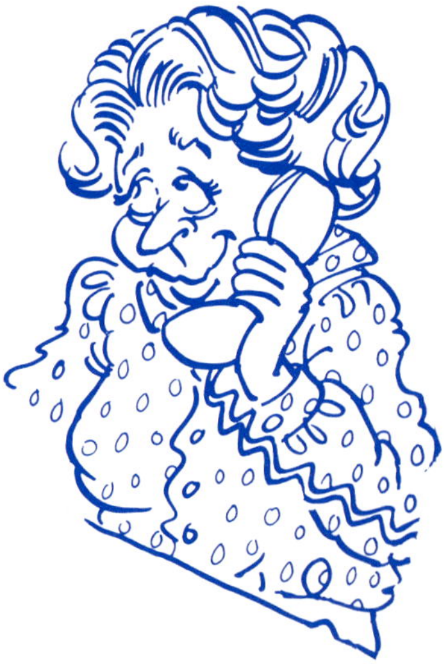

if you think it is urgent, it would be easier for us tomorrow morning', will get a more helpful response from the great majority of patients. If not — well at least you tried! Of course, as we have already seen, some patients may still be angry and you may find it helpful within your groups to discuss some ways in which you cope with this hostility (and even verbal abuse). Coping with hostility is a very stressful part of the receptionist's job and hearing how others manage can help you to learn techniques for managing it.

? How much of an effort do you make to smile, even when dealing with particularly awkward patients?

? How much time do you have for patients? Remember, they are your primary concern.

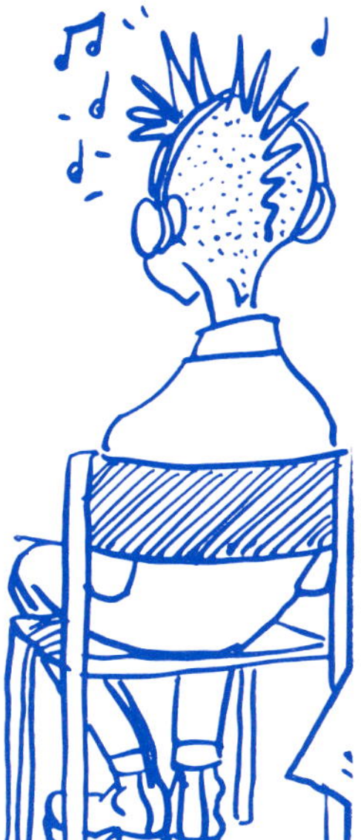

Confidentiality at this point is very important to patients, there are many horror stories of private information being broadcast around a waiting room. Unfortunately many waiting areas and reception points are not designed with the needs of confidentiality in mind. There are often a number of people standing within earshot awaiting attention. If the patient is hard of hearing, and you have to raise your voice, there always seems to be a whole waiting room full of eager listeners. It may be that your doctors are not aware of the problems and that a discussion which might allow the introduction of some structural or organisational changes will help. Some practices have found that they can divide the reception area up into smaller, more private areas. Some have a separate place to which some patients can go to talk. Others have found that music in the waiting room helps. If none of these things is feasible, then the receptionist must do her utmost to avoid a queue. Of course, not everything that is said is confidential, but if you take the trouble to analyse the information you are seeking it is surprising how much is. (We shall pay more attention to this in the section on confidentiality.) It is worth remembering that people who are deaf, hard of hearing, or with language problems, have special needs in terms of confidentiality — we do not usually help understanding by shouting.

A constantly recurring complaint about receptionists is the dislike that so many people have of being asked about the nature of their illness. On the one hand it does seem reasonable that the description of their symptoms or the name of their illness is something that is confidential between them and their doctor. Certainly if this is their view it has to be respected absolutely. On the other hand the receptionist frequently has to make decisions about priorities, about whether patients are fit to wait or about which particular service will be the most appropriate. Trying to do this in the absence of information is difficult. The problem usually arises because the request for further information is not fully explained or tactfully worded so that the patient feels free to decline if necessary. Experienced receptionists will have developed a series of words and phrases that convey these subtleties, such as 'Do you feel you can tell me what the trouble is so that I . . . .' and so on. This is another topic that deserves discussion within your groups.

> ? In what ways do you discover a patient's needs? How would you feel if someone were to ask you the questions you ask patients?

It is very important to record accurately messages that are received. There should be log books to write in — not small and separate pieces of paper. They can easily be lost and leave no record for future reference. For this reason it is also a very good rule to make sure that there is not only a date to the message but a time of receipt as well. Most practices introduce systems of recording incoming messages that take these matters into consideration, indicate the intended recipient of the message, and have a means of showing whether or not the matter has been attended to.

When patients have seen the doctor or nurse, and are leaving the practice, they are usually still thinking about their consultation. They may be trying to remember what has been said, worrying about it, or even worrying about the next thing they have to do. It is very easy for them to 'escape' without making a further appointment so the person working at the reception area has to keep a general watch on the waiting room and on people who are passing to and fro.

> ? How are messages recorded in your practice?
> What techniques do you use when answering the telephone?

COMMUNICATING ON THE TELEPHONE

There are now more telephones per hundred people in Britain than in any other country in Europe. The telephone has become an essential feature of communication between the patient and the surgery and, used intelligently and efficiently, it can be a valuable tool in good patient care, but if mishandled it can be a source of great irritation and potential danger.

Practices try to provide a system that will allow patients to gain access fairly easily. This is sometimes achieved by having a number of lines, by keeping a particular line for outgoing calls or by spreading the load throughout the working day in a variety of different ways. Despite this, useage is so concentrated in the early mornings that it is very often difficult to get through and this may make patients frustrated and irritable. It is not possible to describe a 'best buy' among the many systems available but it is possible to provide some general advice for the receptionist.

The need to give a clear announcement when answering the telephone such as 'Doctors Surgery' is fairly obvious, but not everyone adds a simple phrase such as 'Can I help you?' afterwards, and yet this conveys so much more and takes very little extra time. Remember that a tone of voice can sound either pleasant and welcoming or irritable, and remember to speak slowly at the start of a conversation as people are sometimes a little confused when they are beginning a call, and take some time to adjust. It is good practice to get the name of the caller to start with and if you do not hear it clearly, ask the caller to repeat it. If there is a break in the line later there is then a basis on which to re-establish communication but it is customary for the person who initiated the call to re-make the connection. If it is a patient, try to get the initials or one forename, the surname and the address at the start of the conversation. There should always be pen and paper to hand and this can then be written down. Do not do this on small scraps of paper which can easily get lost but use a proper message book in which the time of receipt of the message can be noted. If it is another doctor or health professional you should try to find out the nature of the call as early as possible so that you can deal with it appropriately. Remember to pitch your voice lower than usual as high notes are more difficult to hear on the telephone, and try to speak very clearly.

A ringing telephone is intrusive, demanding and usually incessant until it is answered. So if you are already engaged in attending to someone when the jangle starts, and it is clear that you are the one who has to lift the receiver, always be thoughtful towards the person you are with. Let the phone give two or three rings, then politely excuse yourself with that person before transferring your attention. It is useful to imagine that the phone is another person, and you would never allow someone just to barge in on a conversation as we sometimes allow a telephone to butt in.

If arrangements have to be made on the telephone they should always depend on positive action; for example, never say 'If you don't hear from me it means that the test is normal.' The correct action would be either to ring and give the result or tell the patient to ring and make a positive enquiry. This way there is no room for doubt. When a message is received which calls for action you cannot deal with yourself, you should make a note of the name, address and telephone number, write the message down and take one of four steps:

1 Transfer the call to someone who can take action
2 Arrange for the caller to be rung back
3 Give a caller a time to be rung back when action can be taken
4 Take and write down a message so that action can be taken

If you are dealing with a patient and cannot attend immediately to the issue you should not leave the caller for long periods without making contact. Every thirty seconds or so say 'I'm sorry to keep you, the doctor is still busy' or some such phrase, and if the patient is in a telephone box, take some immediate action anyway. If the patient is waiting to have a problem dealt with it will be a good opportunity to extract the notes from the files as it should be an absolute rule that the doctor has the notes of patients whenever he is talking to them on the telephone. This is described in greater detail in the chapter on records and forms.

You may sometimes have a patient or relative who talks to you at great length, and you do not have the time to hear them out. In these circumstances you have to be prepared to interrupt them with a question, but try to do it politely. A useful technique is always to use their name before putting the question to them, for example you might say 'Mrs Smith, what exactly was it that you wanted me to ask the doctor?' It is almost impossible to sound rude using this technique. It is always a good plan to repeat the message to the caller before you finish as, in that way, a check is made on its accuracy. You could say 'You want a new prescription for indomethacin and triazolam then Mr Jones?'

It is worthwhile spelling out any words about which you are doubtful. There is an international code that many people are familiar with and it is a good idea to make use of this as much as possible:

A for Andrew
B for Benjamin
C for Charlie
D for David
E for England
F for Frederick
G for George
H for Harry
I for Isaac
J for Jack
K for King
L for Lucy
M for Mary
N for Nelly
O for Oliver
P for Peter
Q for Queenie
R for Robert
S for Sugar
T for Tommy
U for Uncle
V for Victory
W for William
X for Xmas
Y for York
Z for Zebra

Similarly there are standard ways of giving numbers on the telephone. Numbers are always coupled when spoken so that 7123 is spoken as 'seven one — pause — two three'. The figure 0 is spoken as either 'nought' or 'zero' and 00 becomes 'hundred' and 000 becomes 'thousand'.

A pair of numbers is always referred to as 'double' so 714423 becomes 'seven one — pause — double four — pause — two three.'

There is a tendency in a lot of practices to ring a patient back when they wish to speak to the doctor to avoid interrupting the consultation or making a patient hang on too long. It is surprising how grateful patients are for this courtesy but a clear message has to be written in the book about this so that it can be dealt with reliably. This is another good reason why telephone numbers should always be recorded on the outside of the patient's record envelope.

Of course some practices are not in areas where telephones are common to every house and patients may have to walk a long way to find one that has not been vandalized. This will call for a different sort of organisation to that applicable in a more affluent area but any use of the telephone should help communication by being both pleasant and efficient.

Always remember that when someone telephones the doctor it is because they, or a very close relative or friend, are ill, or believe themselves to be ill. It follows that there must be some anxiety or apprehension, which could be manifested by an apparently brusque telephone manner. Do not use your position to chide such callers, or indicate that you do not like their tone of voice. Remain warm, and sound friendly, interested and wanting to help. Let that 'first impression' on the telephone be a good one, and it will almost certainly be reflected in the subsequent visit to the surgery. On the other hand, an unsatisfactory mini-confrontation often takes a long time to be forgotten.

'Yes, you can certainly see the doctor but I am afraid tomorrow morning is the earliest we can book you in', is so much better than 'No, I am afraid you cannot see the doctor today, he is too busy.' There are so many ways in which you can affect the telephone conversation for the better, no matter how great the pressure of work, or how unreasonable the patient might sound. Keep your cool and you keep control.

? What kind of problems have you experienced when using the telephone?

? Have you developed a telephone technique of your own to make people feel more relaxed? Do you use certain phrases or modify the tone of your voice?

COMMUNICATING WITH COLLEAGUES

In the section on the team we consider some of the factors influencing our ability to work with others. They include things like mutual respect,

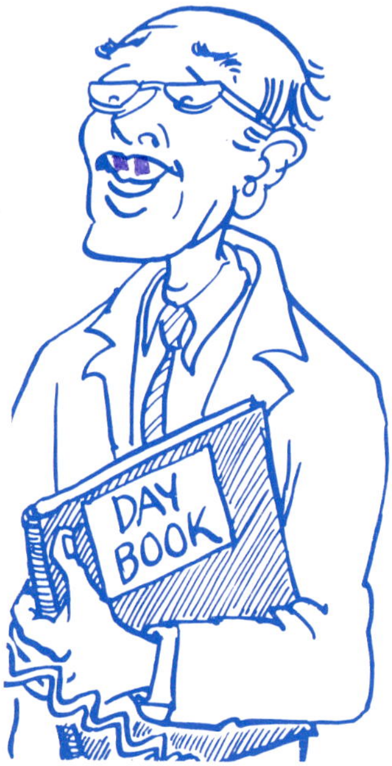

understanding others' roles and so on, but clearly communication is a very important ingredient. Although we work in the practice in quite close physical proximity with each other — the doctor, the nurse and the receptionist are never far removed from each other — we may actually be relatively isolated. The doctor may pass through the office and say 'good morning' and then disappear into his consulting room from which a series of messages may emerge, but he may not be seen again until he collects visits and sets off out again. Similarly the receptionist, busy meeting people in her sphere of activity, may be quite separated from other contacts. The work of each will depend upon the other but this is rarely discussed until problems occur. The separation is not planned or deliberate but is just inherent in the situation. In most practices things are not as bad as this. There is a great deal of informal contact and this is extremely important. There are contacts made as notes are collected, repeat prescriptions are made out, and coffee is taken. All of these contacts help people to get to know each other, appreciate each other's personalities, deal with pressing problems; but there is a need for formal communication as well. Without this sufficient time cannot be set aside for meetings and planning. For example, the receptionist may have difficulties with the telephone arrangements and may wish to propose changes, or the practice nurse may be starting a new clinic. Unless all those involved in the practice get together the effect that it will have on others cannot really be explored. Of course the presence or absence of meetings is not something that a receptionist can decide, but if a meeting is held every effort should be made to attend. It may even be possible to suggest one when it appears to be necessary.

By this time the receptionist should be feeling an important member of an important team. She will know that building up and maintaining understanding and trust with patients and colleagues has to be worked at, and that good communication is vital if this is to be done.

? How much time is set aside in your practice for staff training (in first aid, for instance)?

? How do you communicate with the others working in your practice?

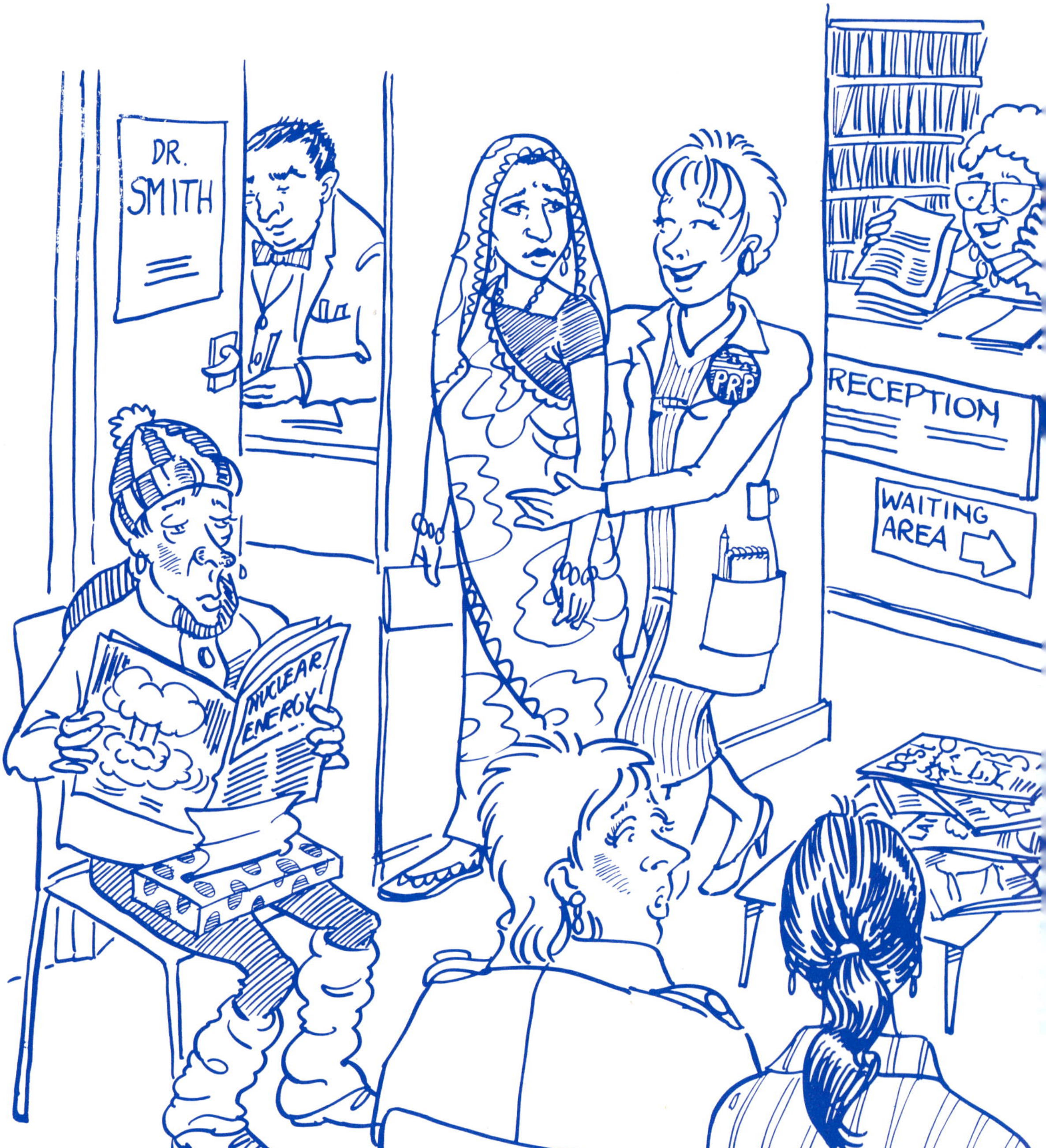

DR. SMITH
RECEPTION
WAITING AREA
PRP
NUCLEAR ENERGY

3 ETHICS AND ETIQUETTE

Confidentiality is such an important constraint upon the behaviour of workers in the health care field that it has a chapter to itself, but there are other important areas of ethical behaviour and etiquette that every receptionist needs to be aware of. The difference between ethics and etiquette is important. Ethics relate to moral principles and are the guiding rules of behaviour. They are all directed towards the benefit of patients and many are now bound up into a code of conduct published by the General Medical Council for doctors and by other bodies for other health professionals. As these bodies all have the responsibility of maintaining the register of those allowed to practice as a doctor, dentist, nurse and so on, the ultimate sanction for those judged to have behaved unethically is the removal of their name from the register and thus the removal of the ability to practice. Etiquette, on the other hand, is concerned with the politenesses of normal behaviour. There are no sanctions for those in breach of etiquette but the 'rules' have been established by custom. They aid communication between professionals and avoid damaging reputations, so they may be said to indirectly benefit patients also. Of course frequently both ethics and etiquette are present at the same time.

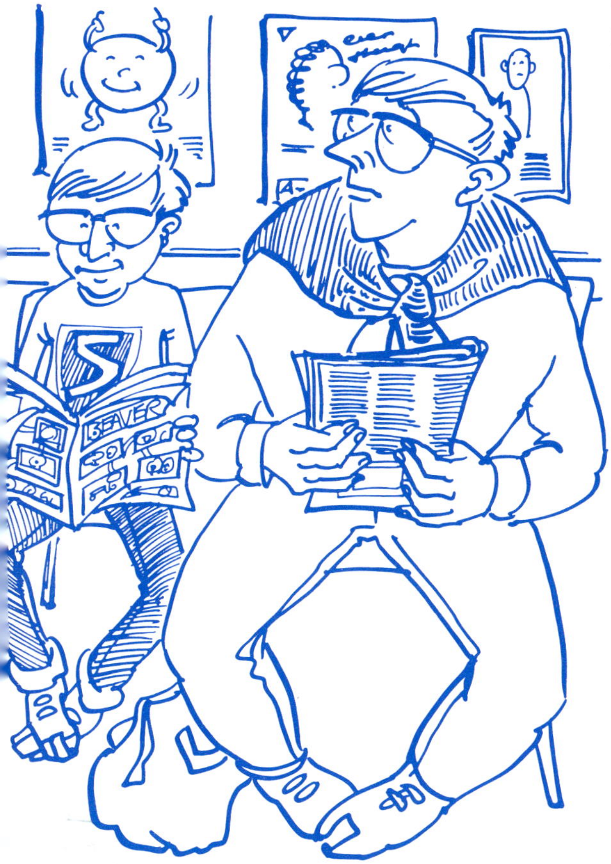

PUBLICITY

Self-advertisement has always been deemed to be unethical. The reason behind this is the belief that false claims to special expertise in achieving a cure will encourage charlatans to advertise and may expose a patient to misleading, and sometimes dangerous, advice. It has always been held that the best source of advice is the patient's own practitioner. However, during the past twenty years matters have become much more complicated. The general public is much better informed medically and is hungry for information. Naturally when they watch television or read articles in the lay press they want to know the authority of the speaker or writer so that they may assess the information they are given. We recognise the importance of people accepting a large measure of responsibility for their own health and that this is best obtained by giving them access to good sources of information. For this reason we have to make a careful distinction between supplying information and self-advertising. This difference is well-illustrated by the recent debate about the production of practice leaflets containing information such as the names of staff, hours of attendance, special facilities available in the surgery and so on. There was little disagreement with the idea of presenting this material to patients who were already registered with a practice and who therefore could not be said to be 'attracted' to the practice by its literature, but the notion of making literature available in libraries and so on was more contentious. In the end it has been agreed that the benefit to the patient of allowing them to make an informed choice of practice outweighed potential disadvantages. It is really the nature of the information that is at issue. What is clearly unethical is any statement implying that the doctor is particularly good or his facilities are better than others. Such a statement would be regarded as self-advertising and unethical. In the same way the doctor's staff has to be very careful not to advertise either when talking to patients in or out of the surgery or chatting to friends. The other side of the coin is related to denigrating the services of other doctor's or dentist's practices or those of other health professionals. It is seldom that one is in full possession of the facts and very easy to jump to conclusions after hearing only half a story. It is unethical to speak disparagingly of another doctor's work or behaviour.

CERTIFICATION

General practitioners are called upon to sign certificates every single working day. These may be forms to allow a patient to claim benefit when

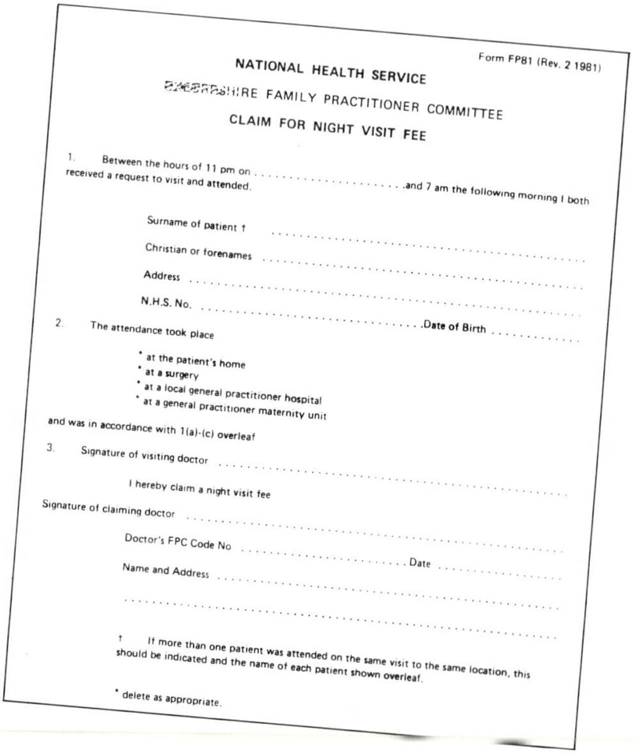

Form FP81 (Rev. 2 1981)

NATIONAL HEALTH SERVICE

[illegible]SHIRE FAMILY PRACTITIONER COMMITTEE

CLAIM FOR NIGHT VISIT FEE

1. Between the hours of 11 pm on .... and 7 am the following morning I both received a request to visit and attended.

Surname of patient † ....

Christian or forenames ....

Address ....

N.H.S. No. .... Date of Birth ....

2. The attendance took place

* at the patient's home
* at a surgery
* at a local general practitioner hospital
* at a general practitioner maternity unit

and was in accordance with 1(a)-(c) overleaf

3. Signature of visiting doctor ....

I hereby claim a night visit fee

Signature of claiming doctor ....

Doctor's FPC Code No .... Date ....

Name and Address ....

....

....

† If more than one patient was attended on the same visit to the same location, this should be indicated and the name of each patient shown overleaf.

* delete as appropriate.

off sick or they may be applications for passports, when a doctor has to certify that the applicant is known to him. They may be claims for services given, such as making a visit at night or attending a temporary resident. The General Medical Council and the courts take a very serious view indeed of false certification even when it is brought about by carelessness and is clearly not an attempt to defraud. It is important that a receptionist recognises that when a doctor signs a form which certifies that he has seen a patient, he must actually have seen him or her, and this has to be carefully explained to the patient, who might otherwise just think that everyone is trying to be officious.

CHAPERONING

Doctors and dentists are particularly liable to accusations of sexual misconduct with patients. This is partly due to the vulnerability of some patients, who may be psychologically disturbed, and partly due to the close relationship that a doctor has to establish with a patient if he is to be able to help them. Sometimes accusations are the result of words said or things that are properly done but which have been misinterpreted. The complete safeguard for the doctor is to have a third party chaperoning the consultation. This has to be done discreetly and unobtrusively for a third party at

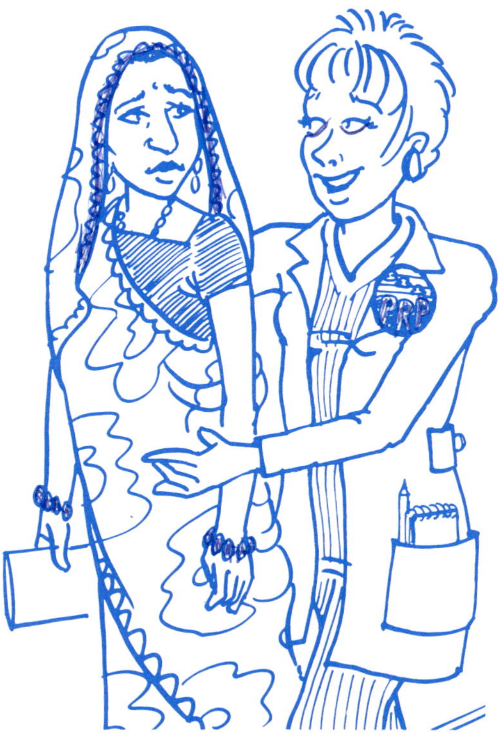

a consultation always introduces an extra dimension to what transpires and on a number of occasions their presence is unacceptable to the patient. Often however it is not possible to have a chaperone present: the speed at which work takes place, the doctor's home visiting list, the fact that some patients require an examination whilst others do not, all tend to make it impractical for a chaperone to be present. When it is *not* possible for a chaperone to be present during an examination one should always be within earshot; the sensitive receptionist will fill this role without being asked.

? What effects do you think a chaperone's presence has on the consultation?

? How does this affect confidentiality between doctor and patient?

ACCEPTING PATIENTS

It is obviously important for patients that their treatment is not being provided by more than one doctor at any one time. If this were to happen patients might be given conflicting and confusing advice or receive two forms of treatment which are incompatible or even dangerous. Of course, at times, it might seem to patients that this removes from them the ability to choose between different advice from different doctors. This is true to some extent, but on balance it seems that the dangers of dual treatment are the greatest, so the practice of assigning responsibility to one general practitioner exists. Consultants will normally only accept patients who have been referred to them by a general practitioner. Then, having dealt with the problem for which referral took place, they will return the patient to the care of the general practitioner. In this way a consultant will not refer a patient to another consultant for a different condition without going back to the general practitioner, nor will they treat a patient for another condition which is unrelated to the problem they have been consulted about. Occasionally these rules are not followed but such behaviour is generally unethical and in theory may place the patient in some jeopardy. In the same way no general practitioner will treat the patient of another general practitioner except in a case of emergency or when the patient is away from home, or when, in special circumstances, a patient is referred to him by the G.P. for a second opinion. In all these cases he will return the patient to his own doctor's care and will send a clinical note to the responsible doctor as soon as possible. This explains why, when a patient wishes to change his doctor, he either has to get consent from his present doctor, or wait for two weeks before receiving treatment, though these rules are currently under review.

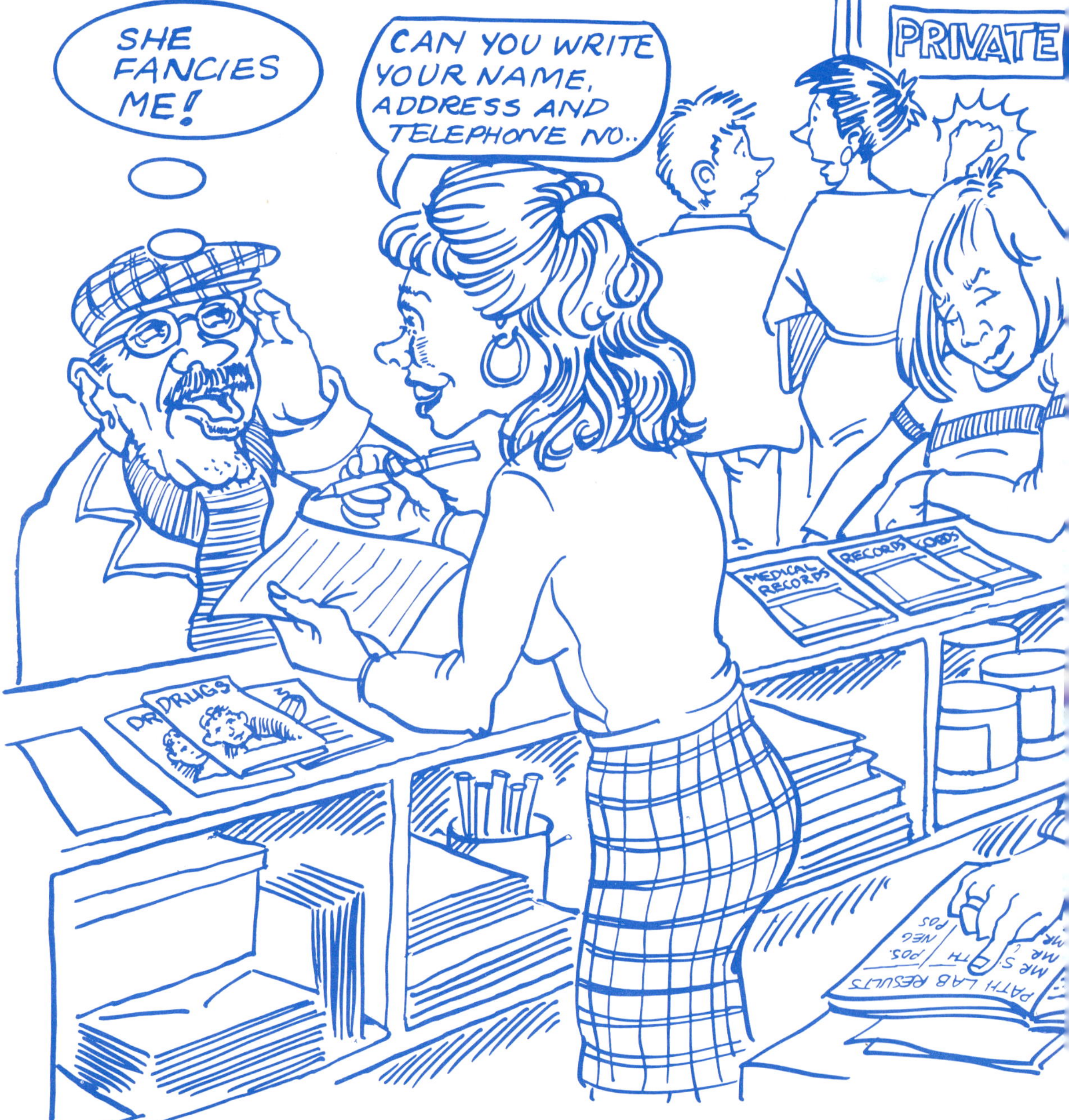
SHE FANCIES ME!
CAN YOU WRITE YOUR NAME, ADDRESS AND TELEPHONE NO..
PRIVATE
DRUGS
MEDICAL RECORDS
RECORDS
PATH LAB RESULTS
POS.
NEG

4

CONFIDENTIALITY

The notion that information a doctor obtains during the course of his work from his patient should be confidential is as old as medicine itself. The Hippocratic Oath, written by a group of doctors who studied under Hippocrates on the island of Cos in the fifth century B.C., contained the following sentence – 'Whatsoever I see or hear, in the lives of men, which ought not to be spoken abroad, I shall not divulge, as reckoning that all such should be kept secret.'

It seems a simple and straightforward idea and is designed both to protect the patient and to encourage other patients to give information which might be important in making the diagnosis or in deciding on the management of an illness. When most medical care was of a relatively simple nature and involved just one doctor and one patient it was easy to apply, but today care has become much more complex. Many doctors are often involved in the care of the patient and they have a need to share information. Other health care workers such as nurses, secretaries, physiotherapists and so on may be involved and may need information about the patient. Because of this confidential facts can leak out accidentally. Relatives and colleagues of a patient may find their lives much affected by his illness and might claim that they should also be a party to knowledge that will allow them to plan matters for the benefit of the patient or for other people. Information is needed for people to obtain mortgages or life insurances, certificates to enable people to have shotguns or to fly gliders, to drive heavy goods vehicles or obtain parking permits. Usually the consent of the patient is sought before this information is transmitted to a third party, but in these days of electronic communication it may be difficult to be certain where exactly the passage of information ends. Nevertheless, although special circumstances may lead to some modification from time to time, the cardinal rule exists that information learnt about a patient by a doctor in the course of his work must never be passed on to a third party without the patient's consent. This rule applies equally to any other health care professional involved with the patient. We shall now go on to consider the various points in primary care where accidental

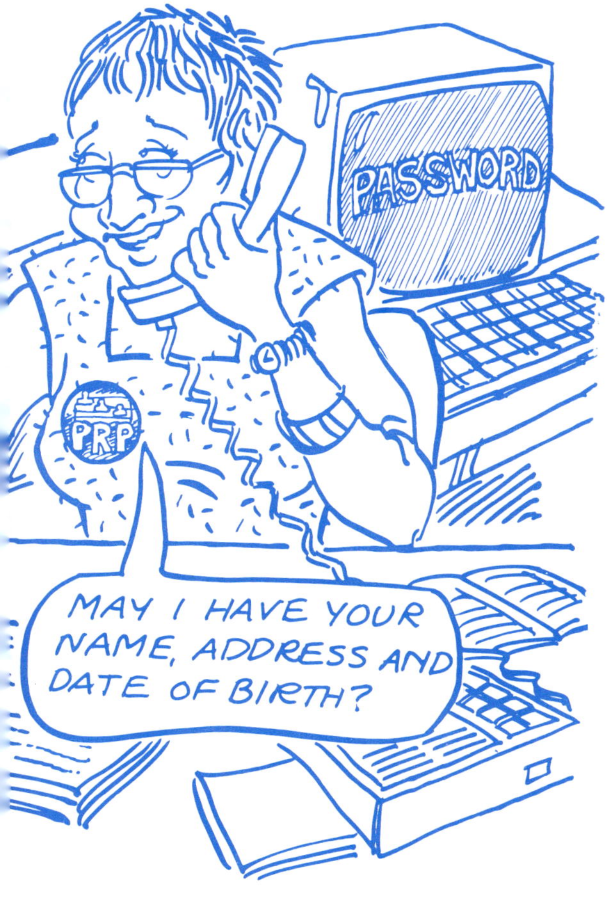

breaches of confidentiality may occur and consider what steps are necessary to lessen the risk. It may be useful to consider each of these in your group work with your own practice in mind.

THE RECEPTION DESK AND WAITING ROOM

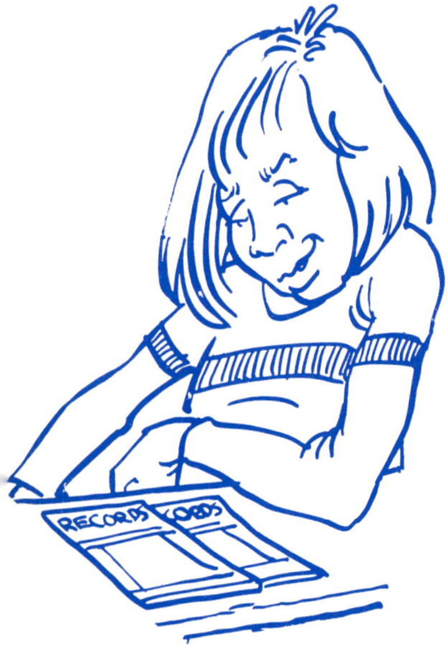

Reception areas vary enormously in design and structure. Some practices have a single 'hatch' which will accommodate one patient talking to a receptionist while a queue builds up behind him. Others have a long desk with a number of receptionists, who may be separated from each other to restrict sound. Reception areas will, at some times of the day, have large numbers of people wanting attention and at other times will be quiet. Obviously the ability to maintain confidentiality will be influenced greatly both by the layout and the degree of activity, and these are to some extent outside the receptionist's control. A skilled receptionist will, however, develop techniques for shielding the patient. This will be done partly by being careful about what is said, particularly in earshot of the waiting room, and partly by having an area where the patient is able to discuss matters with the receptionist in privacy. It is not possible to explain to a patient, for example, how to collect a mid-stream specimen of urine, without such an arrangement, nor is it possible to get an indication of the patient's problems so that appropriate urgency can be applied without being able to make private enquiries. This is particularly so if the patient is deaf or has difficulty in understanding and needs a loud tone of voice or repeated explanations.

This question of asking a patient what is wrong with them is a matter of great contention. The receptionist has to decide whether a patient is fit enough to sit in the waiting room or should be helped by a nurse. Many patients, however, feel annoyed at being asked to divulge medical matters to anyone other than the doctor, especially when they have spent a lot of time plucking up enough courage even to tell the doctor. There are ways of doing it. A bald question such as 'What is wrong with you?' is likely to produce some very unhelpful comments and antagonistic feelings in patients. A question such as 'Are you able to tell me what the problem is?' is a softer approach, and if expanded by some such remark as 'so that we can arrange the best place for you to be seen', is completely acceptable to most. Remember, in this area the customer is always right, and if the patient demonstrates any hesitance or reluctance to give information this must be accepted with a smile. It is, after all, his inalienable right to choose what information he wants to give and to whom. Another problem that can arise at the reception area concerns people coming on behalf of a patient. It is extremely common for relatives and friends to offer to help a patient. by collecting forms or letters on his behalf, or by asking for the results of tests. Strictly speaking no-one but the patient is entitled to this information and this rule should be applied. Indeed girls under 16 requesting contraceptive advice are entitled to confidentiality, though the doctor should make every attempt to persuade her to tell her parents. It applies to mothers and children, to husbands and wives, to employers and employees, and a breach of this rule, even by something seemingly harmless such as telling the husband the result of a pregnancy test, can cause the most serious trouble. Of course any rule has to be applied with some measure of flexibility and common sense and there are bound to be occasional exceptions. The vast majority of people will understand being told that you cannot pass on this information, for they themselves might be the patient next time and will feel secure in the knowledge of high standards of confidentiality.

If written material which is confidential is passed over the desk to anyone other than the patient, it must be sealed in an addressed envelope.

> ? What techniques do you use to find out how pressing a patient's need is without causing embarrassment?

THE TELEPHONE

The proportion of houses with a telephone increases yearly and the number of telephone requests for information goes up in parallel. Most of the rules about confidentiality that apply to the reception desk apply with equal force to the telephone, but there is the added complication that you cannot always tell that the person on the telephone is who they claim to be. The difficulties that can arise from asking the patient the nature of the problem are highly relevant to telephone enquiries. Many are requests for visits and the patient may, rightly or wrongly, believe that the receptionist is making the decision about the need for a visit at all. It is certainly not the place of the receptionist to present the patient with a detailed series of questions. The only relevant questions relate to the address and to the degree of urgency attributed by the person requesting the visit. Remember that telephone lines occasionally get crossed, and that even one side of a telephone call overheard by other patients can seriously breach confidentiality.

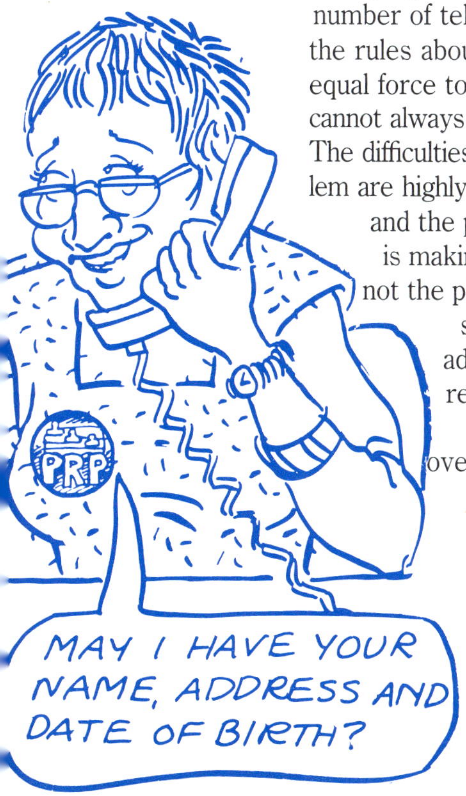

LETTERS AND REPORTS

No information about a patient should be transmitted in writing unless the patient has given his or her consent. If a letter is the result of a consultation with a patient, such as a letter of a referral to a consultant, it can be assumed that consent was given at the time of the consultation. In all other respects, whether the request for information is from another doctor or from a lay person, formal signed consent to divulge information should be received and should be kept in the notes thereafter. Anything else, for example requests from solicitors or doctors working for insurance companies, must be refused until written consent has been obtained.

Letters and reports which give information must be treated in the same confidential manner as those which request information and must not be left about where they can be seen by third parties. Care has also to be taken about passing information from a third party to a fourth. For example, a hospital specialist may write to a doctor with a report about a patient and feel aggrieved if his opinion is passed on to another person without his consent. It is a difficult area, but there is one hard and fast rule: nothing, however trivial, should be done to breach confidentiality unless there is no doubt that the patient will benefit from such a breach in confidentiality — and the patient is usually the best judge of that. Even this cannot be a totally rigid rule, for very occasionally the doctor has to consider that the public good overrides the individual patient's needs. For example, a driver who has epileptic fits and does not want the licensing authority to know, or the doctor has evidence relating to a serious crime which the patient does not want the police to know. These are rare but serious occasions and the doctor has to make the decision since he bears the ultimate responsibility. There is only one circumstance when the rule of confidentiality *never* applies and that is when the doctor is ordered by a court to make a disclosure.

RECORDS

The records of the patient are the ultimate repository of confidential information about the patient. The National Health records are the property of the Secretary of State for Health but it has been held in several cases that opinions expressed within the notes are the property of the person who recorded them. It is very important that records are kept secure. Ideally they should be kept in lockable cabinets or at least in a lockable room. The receptionist needs to take care over this matter and make certain that no-one can see the records of any patient except those entitled to. Where care is shared by a number of people, such as nurses, health visitors or social workers, the receptionist should ensure that the doctor has given consent for another person to see the notes. This may be a

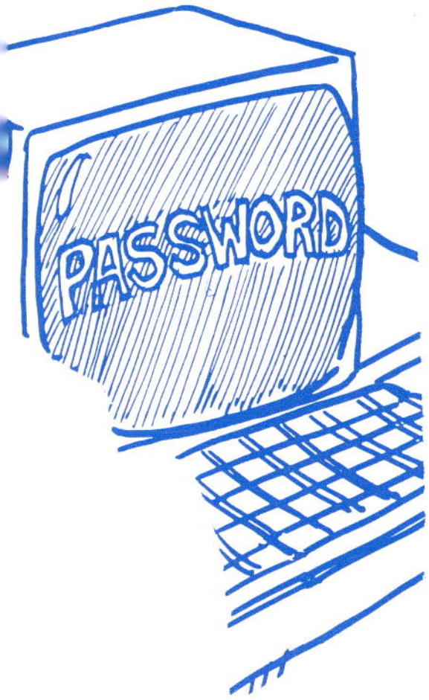

blanket approval, say in the case of a practice nurse, or may refer only to a single sheet of records, but the receptionist must be sure what is meant. Some records are now being kept on computers and this raises other issues. In general computer-held material is at least as confidential as a paper record. 'Confidentiality', in relation to computers is not the same as the word 'security' applied to computers. Whereas confidentiality relates to the privacy of information, security relates to the ability to store information, without risk of its being accidentally erased. In fact, with care, computer held information should be more confidential since it is possible to write programmes which allow different people different levels of access. For example, it is possible to give a doctor access via the computer to all the information in the patients notes, whereas the medical secretary only has access to identification material (name and address, date of birth and so on).

There are two problem areas. First, computers can be connected together so that they can 'talk' to each other. Thus communications received in confidence, for example when a patient has consented to medical details going to an insurance company, may be transmitted too widely, say to another insurance company or to a potential employer. Second, in transmitting material which is not confidential a breach of confidentiality may inadvertantly occur. For example, in a research project it may be agreed to transmit all the medical information related to pregnant patients except names and addresses, but if there is only one patient who has triplets, or one patient aged thirty-seven years who had a baby, a deduction can be made that will breach confidentiality. The Data Protection Act, which requires users of computers storing personal data about other people to register and to obey certain rules, is designed to protect people as far as possible. In spite of all this the commonest way in which confidentiality is breached in practice is the spoken word. We all live in communities with our patients. People ask 'How is Mrs Jones?' and in the shop or at the party it is tempting to reply using knowledge obtained in the course of work. What is, for most people, normal social conversation and friendly gossip becomes quite unacceptable and unethical behaviour and all health professionals are at risk. Confidentiality as well as freedom is only guarded by eternal vigilance.

? How important is confidentiality?

How would you feel if the nature of your illness were known to all your friends?

? How you would you feel if a member of the practice staff refused to tell you what your husband/son/daughter were suffering from?

5 THE NATIONAL HEALTH SERVICE

In this section we shall consider some aspects of the structure of the health service. Most receptionists will already have some knowledge of parts of this but it is helpful to have an idea about the general concepts governing the system within which we work. The years between the two world wars were the period when most of the debate about a national health service took place. The hospitals were nearly bankrupt and only part of the population was covered by an insurance scheme. Even whilst the war was going on, and it was far from certain that we should win, plans were being produced, and in 1946 the National Health Service Act was passed. The essential feature of the Act that made it different from all that had preceded it was that now treatment would be available to all and not just those who had paid contributions. Although it has been modified and the service has been reorganised several times, the paramount governing principle remains the same today.

There are three arms to the health services. The hospital services look after patients who require in-patient or out-patient specialist advice. Primary care services, both medical and dental, as well as sight testing and pharmaceutical services, are looked after by another branch, and services concerned with environment and infectious disease control have yet another separate structure.

Here we are concerned with primary care services. Primary care is that provided to patients as a result of first contact with health care. Mostly it is the responsibility of the family doctor service but there are two other services which for special reasons, confidentiality and urgency, form part of primary care but are actually managed by the hospital. These are sexually transmitted disease services and accident and emergency services. Apart from these two services, which can be seen as special, and family planning, which is organised in yet another way, no-one can gain access to medical care without going through the family doctor system.

FAMILY PRACTITIONER COMMITTEE

In England and Wales this system is organised by Family Practitioner Committees, in Scotland by Health Boards and in Northern Ireland by Health and Social Services Boards. But in spite of these differences, and the use of some different documentation and record forms in the various countries, the principles of the service are the same in any part of the United Kingdom.

There are more than 30,000 general practitioners looking after a population of nearly fifty-nine million, so on average there are about 1,900 patients per doctor. This figure may vary from a few hundred in remote rural areas and some city areas to 3,000 in other places but most have about 2,000 patients. Whereas at the start of the Health Service most doctors worked single-handed and were assisted only by their wives, today more than eighty per cent are in a group practice and there are about 10,000 practices into which the general practitioners are grouped in the U.K.

The Family Practitioner Committee, or its counterpart in Scotland and N. Ireland, has various tasks in relation to primary medical care. It administers the doctor's contract and pays him although, unlike the hospital doctor, the G.P. is not salaried. It maintains the register of patients and may use this for organising certain services. The Family Practitioner Committee holds two lists. The first is an alphabetical list of all the patients in the area for which it is responsible and the second list shows which patients are allocated to which individual doctors and practices. These lists were held manually but now most are computerised and can be used for other purposes. For example now that F.P.C.s undertake recall for cervical cytology, the register of patients, together with their addresses and birth dates, forms an essential part of health care administration.

The general practitioner is not an employee of the National Health Service in the same way as the hospital doctor. General practice was not 'nationalised' in 1946 as were the hospital services, the coal mines, the railways and the steel industry. General practitioners were invited to enter into a contract with the Health Service for the care of those patients who registered with them. An analogy is a firm of builders who are constructing a housing estate and wish to install a proper electrical system in each house. They may not have their own electricians so they will sub-contract work to electricians who will carry out the service and, providing it is carried out within the range of cost, quality and time specified, the arrangements are left to the sub-contractors. There was nothing new about this idea being applied in health care for it was only an extension of an insurance principle that had applied to certain groups of workers for a long time and had been gradually extending since the First World War. What was new was that now it would apply to everybody.

Since the general practitioner is an independent contractor and not an employee of the National Health Service, one could be expected to ask at this stage — How then is the general practitioner remunerated? Quite uniquely!

Clearly the general practitioner is remunerated in a totally different manner from his hospital-based colleague, the hospital doctor being paid as a direct employee and on a particular scale of salary through house doctor, registrar and consultant gradings, under the Pay As You Earn system.

For historical reasons, some of which have been set out in this chapter, the general practitioner's remuneration is complex. In the main, the general practitioner is paid in the form of fees and allowances which come to him via the Family Practitioner Committee. These fees and allowances fall in to various categories and are set out in detail in the 'Red Book' (Statement of

Fees and Allowances), and often can be found in a more simple form in the medical press.

The categories are summarised below:

Basic practice allowance
Capitation fees
Item of service fees
Other allowances and payments from FPC
NHS income separate from FPC

If we look at the various components of this financial structure it will clarify the relationship between the doctor and the health authority and it will explain the reasons behind a lot of the things receptionists have to do in the surgery.

BASIC PRACTICE ALLOWANCE

These allowances represent a fixed part of the doctor's pay, which is needed as a minimum for running a practice of over 1000 patients. On top of this basic practice allowance there can be additions for leave, group practice, seniority, vocational training, out of hours service, for practising in a designated area, and for employing an assistant.

There are of course qualifying conditions for these allowances and again one can find them set out in detail in the 'Red Book' – see page 39.

CAPITATION FEES

The list of patients registered with the doctor is held by the F.P.C. (or its equivalent in Scotland and Northern Ireland). The doctor is paid a quarter of his capitation fee for each patient every three months. Because patients who are elderly need more services, a doctor practising in an area with a high proportion of elderly people may not be able to look after as many patients as a doctor with a list of mainly middle-aged people. So an increased capitation fee is paid for people over sixty-five years of age and more for those over seventy-five years of age. There are patients who need care and who are not on the doctor's list, people who are either temporarily resident in the area or who require emergency treatment and these have to be dealt with in a different manner.

There are three reasons for maintaining the accuracy of the list. First, the patient's records must be transferred as quickly as possible when a patient changes doctor. Second, if the details on the list are not accurate it becomes very difficult for the Health Authority to communicate with the patient about, say, preventive care. Third, the list forms an important element of the practice income. A patient is of course only allowed to register with one doctor and that patient will then expect to receive all their care from that doctor or his practice under the National Health Service. Fees may not be charged to that patient except for certain services which are not part of health care, such as filling in insurance certificates, or examining for fitness to work as a heavy goods vehicle driver or to hang-glide.

What are the three 'wings' of the National Health Service?

ITEM OF SERVICE FEES

We shall see in the section on 'Records and Forms' how payments are dealt with in general practice. Here we are looking at the concepts and principles behind these payments. The registered list enables capitation fees to be paid. In order to encourage some clinical activities to take place a fee is paid for certain items of service above and beyond this. The principle behind this is that preventive medicine needs a special boost in order to compete with curative medicine, so care such as immunisation, contraception, cervical cytology and maternity medical services are rewarded in this way. It is probable that this form of remuneration will increase as it is capable of being accurately monitored.

Can you give examples of the services for which a patient may be expected to pay a fee?

OTHER ALLOWANCES AND PAYMENTS FROM F.P.C.

A number of other fees and allowances are payable by the F.P.C. There is a fairly extensive list and the following are one or two examples:

Training grant
Dispensing payments
Fees for reports to Regional Medical Officers
Expenses for doctors attendance at postgraduate meetings

N.H.S. INCOME SEPARATE FROM F.P.C.

General practitioners may undertake sessional work for hospitals or social services or perhaps lectures to health authority staff etc. These fees will be paid directly from the health authority with national insurance, tax and superannuation possibly being deducted. A careful and detailed record of all these payments must be kept. Over and above N.H.S. income, the general practitioner may be paid for medical services requested from a wide variety of sources — private insurance medicals, legal issues would be two examples.

Such fees are usually paid at rates agreed with the British Medical Association, so an up to date schedule of fees is needed.

An abbreviated version of 'recommended fees' can often be found in the medical press.

PREMISES AND STAFF

The Family Practitioner Committee has responsibilities in relation to both these topics. It has to satisfy itself that the standard of premises in which patients are seen is adequate. It does more than this, it helps doctors in the planning and construction of new buildings and in the conversion or adaptation of old buildings. In this way more than eighty per cent of practices have been rehoused in the past few years.

In 1966 a revolution took place in the way that practices were encouraged to employ staff to assist in patient care. From that time on doctors who worked together in groups were entitled to employ up to two full-time staff per doctor, to be engaged in specified duties such as the reception of patients, and to receive a repayment of seventy per cent of their salary and all their National Insurance payments. This was a huge encouragement and there has been a steady increase in the numbers of such staff at work since then.

DISTRIBUTION OF DOCTORS

When the health service began there were areas of the country which were short of doctors and other areas with a surplus. Over the years, health care planning, together with an increased intake of newly qualified doctors, has meant that the average list size has dropped by nearly 1,000 patients per doctor and that the unequal distribution has been largely corrected. There are still a few areas short of doctors such as in very rural areas where an incentive payment in the form of a salary is needed to help the doctor start or maintain his practice but, by and large, fair distribution is assured. In some city areas a few patients have difficulties getting on to a chosen practice list simply because city-centre doctors' lists are bulging. Where this is so the F.P.C. will provide a patient with a doctor as close to the patient's home as possible.

In 1946 over eighty per cent of doctors worked single-handed. Now more than eighty per cent work in partnership. This has been actively encouraged by successive governments by an additional payment made to doctors who work in groups. The arguments for group practices are that they are more cost-effective: a piece of equipment such as an E.C.G. machine or additional staff can be used more efficiently by a group than by an individual. Furthermore the ability of patients to share views with doctors and have access to a variety of doctors young and old, male and female, is enhanced. Lastly, the isolation of the single-handed doctor is removed. Perhaps one obvious disadvantage is that of size. We now often recognise this in other situations such as shops, factories or hotels, biggest does not necessarily mean best. The biggest organisation may be the most impersonal and be the most obstructive to good communication. This has to be consciously worked at in a group practice and within a team.

? In what ways can continuity of care for patients be assisted?

? In what type of practice do you work?

What are the extra benefits of group practices?

THE 'RED BOOK'

There are other duties of F.P.C.s, such as investigating complaints from patients and distributing information to doctors but they are beyond the scope of this section. More detail can be discovered in the The Statement of Fees and Allowances — the 'Red Book'. This is a ring folder in which all the regulations are set out. It is important that it is kept up to date by the insertion of amendments and additions as they arrive. It is worth looking through the 'Red Book' quickly to see what it is about.

You may think it useful in your groups to consider the relationship between your practice and the F.P.C. Many F.P.C.s welcome visits from the practice staff and can advise on the easiest way to maintain efficient communication.

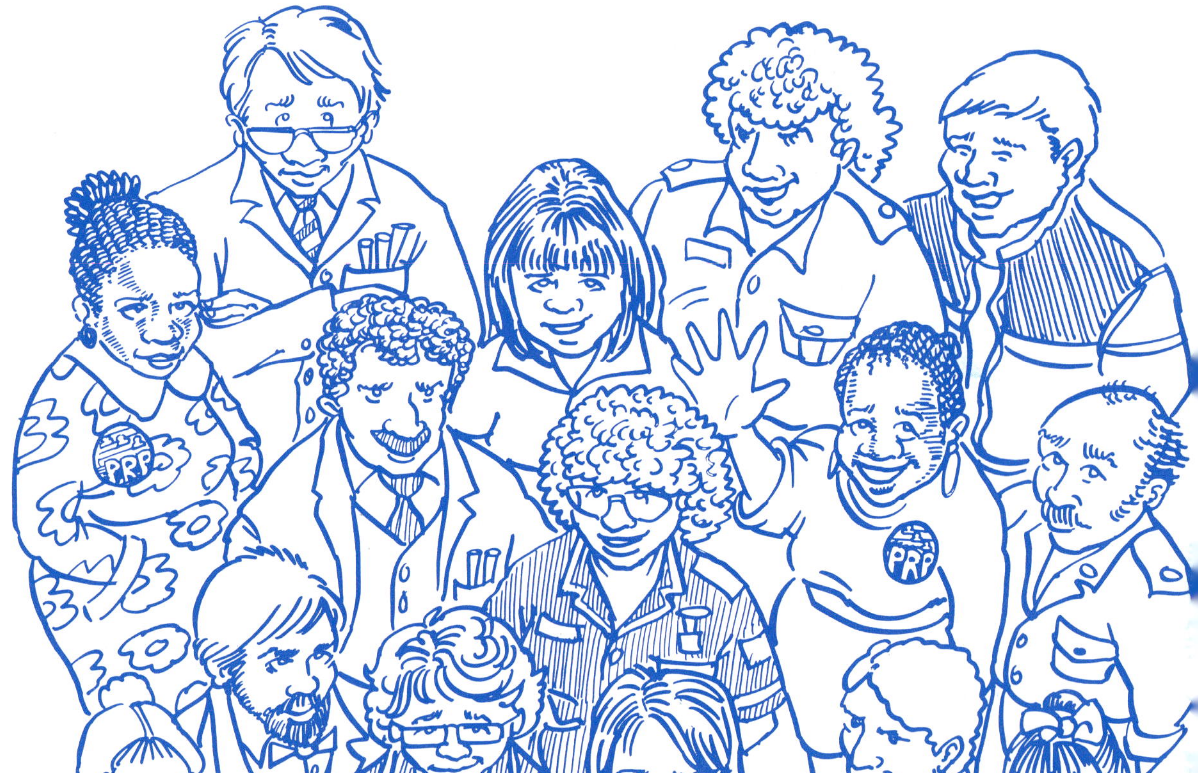
PRP
PRP
PRP

6

THE HEALTH TEAM

As medical care has become more complex, the variety of skills required to help has multiplied and this has led to the concept of a number of people working together as a team. One study showed that in nearly forty per cent of consultations a general practitioner required the help of some other health care worker. There are however a lot of problems concerned with team work. Sometimes valuable members of the team are not included. For example, we may not be aware of the existence of a home care service to help with the terminally ill so we may fail to recruit it. Sometimes there may be a breakdown in communications leading either to overlap — several people doing the same task — or to an actual gap where the service is not provided at all. At other times there may be differences of opinion or personality clashes and inevitably when this happens it is the patient who suffers. It is perhaps incorrect to talk about *the* team. There are a whole number of different teams involved in the care of some patients that interact with each other from time to time. There are also subsets of teams so that the practice team will have within it a nursing subset consisting perhaps of a practice nurse, a district nurse, a health visitor and a midwife. They have to relate to an administrative subset consisting of a practice manager, a secretary, receptionists and filing clerks, who have a different sphere of interest. What are the factors that make for good team-work? The answer to this question allows us to develop our place in the team.

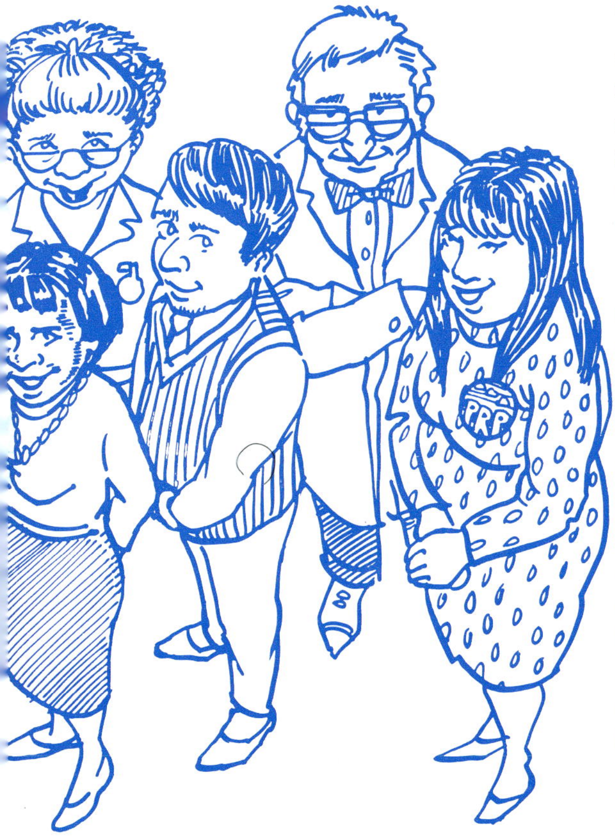

CREDIBILITY

The dictionary definition of this is 'worthy of belief' and that is extremely important to us in all sorts of fields. We need to have self-respect and to have a personal belief in the value of what we are trying to do — that applies to our professional lives as well as our private lives. The reason people go on courses is because they have this belief and want to enhance their skills and their usefulness at work. But there is more to it than just self-respect because we need to have the respect of others. If they too believe in the value of what we are trying to do then they will use our skills. It is possible for us to respect some jobs such as those of computer programmer or magnetic resonance technician, because we don't know what they do; the mystique surrounding the position seems to make them believable. But if we want to work with them we need to know what skills they have and the way in which they may be brought to bear on particular problems. So it is important to know about other people's jobs for them to be 'credible' and for us to be able to use their skills to the maximum advantage of the patients. One of the objectives of this part of the book will be to set out the roles of various members of teams with whom you come into contact thus helping to establish their credibility.

COMMUNICATION

It seems so obvious that good communication is a requirement for a team to work well that it is hardly worth stating, but it only takes a moment or two of reflection about the problems that arise in a surgery to recognise our failings in this respect.

— Mr Jones comes out of hospital on Friday afternoon with a discharging wound and a small collection of tablets. His wife rings up on Thursday morning 'in a state'. He has run out of tablets, the dressings are smelly, and she doesn't know what to do except that she would like to kick someone!

Did the failing start with the hospital? Whose fault could it have been? The ward clerk? The ward sister? The house surgeon? Did it start in the practice with the receptionist or the G.P.? Was it the responsibility of the Community Nurses to know about the patient?

Of course when things work smoothly, which they usually do, we rarely hear about any problems. It only requires one episode, however, like the example quoted, to undo a lot of good work. That is why we must pay particular attention to good communication.

> ? What methods of communication do you have with other members of the health team? Do you have formal meetings with other members of the team?

CONFIDENTIALITY

This has been dealt with in greater detail already. To sum up: as team-work develops and more people get involved in any situation, confidentiality becomes a more important issue. It depends upon mutual trust between the members of a team and is enhanced by keeping a team fairly small. There is another side of the coin to beware of. It is possible for a team to become so close that they feel all sorts of highly confidential information about a patient can be flipped about within the team without having any mandate from the patient to do so. It is important to share information but only when that sharing is necessary for patient care.

We can at this point identify the characteristics of good teamwork. They are:

1. There is a common purpose shared by all the members of the team
2. Every member of the team understands his or her function and those of the fellow members
3. Team members share information and resources and have common responsibility

How does your practice agree the tasks to be set? Are you certain about your role?

Do you know what the roles are of other members of the team with whom you work closely? How are decisions made within your team?

Does the team follow up decisions that are made? How does your team deal with conflict?

Does the team work efficiently? Is morale high in your team? If not, why not?

In the next section we shall briefly explore the roles of some of the key workers with whom you may be involved. They include the community nursing sisters, health visitors, the practice nurses, midwives, social workers, community psychiatric nurses and the home care team.

COMMUNITY NURSING SISTERS

These used to be known as District Nurses because they worked on a geographical basis looking after the nursing needs of patients in their own homes. They are now more often than not attached to a single practice and work with the patients belonging to that practice, or perhaps the patients of two smaller practices. Practice attachment gives them a chance to work more closely in a team with other staff but has the disadvantage of spreading their work over a very wide area. Occasionally these nurses work in the treatment room of the practice. They are employed by the health authority and are fully trained nurses who have experience in hospitals before coming to work in the community. They are involved in traditional nursing duties such as treating people who are ill at home with heart failure, acute chest conditions, terminal illness or, increasingly, after early discharge from hospital. These patients may require wound dressings, attention to bowels, prevention of bed sores and so on, and their relatives at home will gain great support from being taught how to help the patient themselves or just by knowing that someone will be coming in regularly.

HEALTH VISITORS

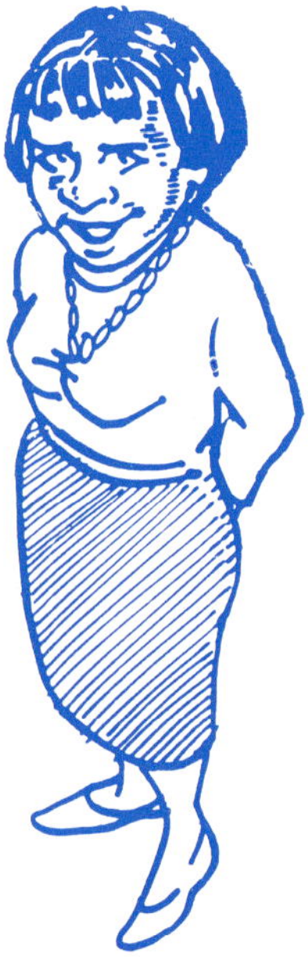

The health visitor is a trained nurse with a post-registration qualification, employed by the District Health Authority, and working mainly as a member of the primary health care team. The training of health visitors is rooted in the promotion of health and they learn to recognise the effects of psychological, social, economic and environmental factors on health and this enables them to fulfil their role in health education and the prevention of disease.

Although health visitors are concerned with all age groups, they have a special responsibility for the under-fives. New-born babies are visited in their own homes, and parents advised on matters of child health and development. Emphasis is given to the need for immunisation and the value of attending a child health clinic. They are also concerned with other vulnerable groups such as the elderly, the physically and mentally handicapped, single parents, and families under stress. In addition they may be involved in the provision of health surveillance programmes and research, in which case an age/sex register or other form of data base is particularly helpful.

PRACTICE NURSES

These form a rapidly growing group of health care workers and represent one way by which health services are changing to meet new challenges. They are employed by the practice and do most of their work within the treatment room. They are usually fully trained nurses who have had experience in hospital and other fields before taking up practice work. Practice nurses are employed in traditional work in the treatment room such as applying dressings, giving injections, syringing ears and removing sutures. The range of their activity is changing to include the shared care of groups of patients with chronic diseases such as hypertension, diabetes and asthma and involvement in preventive work such as taking cervical smears, breast and blood pressure screening and the immunisation of adults. Practice nurses are beginning to use some of the tools that were traditionally used only by the doctor such as ophthalmoscopes, stethoscopes, auroscopes and vaginal speculae. Further important extensions of their work involve counselling, listening and reassuring.

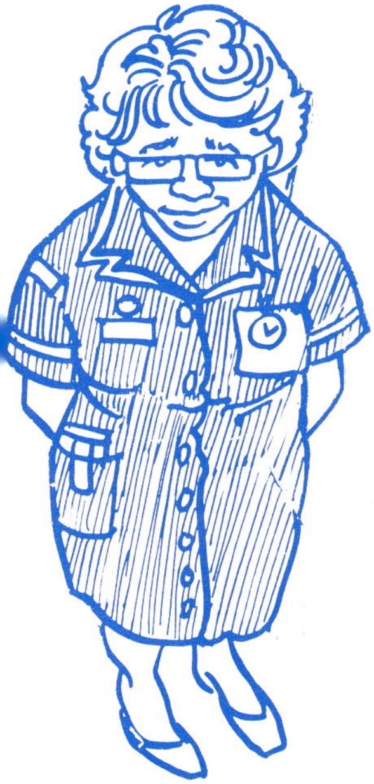

MIDWIVES

Midwives have a central role in the care of pregnant women. They are fully trained nurses who have then completed a prolonged midwifery course. They are employed by the health authority and they form part of the team with hospital obstetricians, general practitioners and health visitors concerned with antenatal care, antenatal preparation, intrapartum care, delivery, and postpartum care of the mother and infant. They run antenatal clinics sometimes with doctors, and conduct normal deliveries in hospital and occasionally in the home. They are also very much involved in the postpartum care of mothers discharged home early after delivery.

SOCIAL WORKERS

In about one in five consultations a doctor becomes involved in discussions and advice about personal relationships, work, social benefits, social support or other financial matters. These are important features of primary care, but just as the doctor will want to call on the special skills of nurses for some problems so he will want to use a social worker's skills in the issues listed above.

If, for example, a young unmarried mother is taken ill the problem extends beyond the immediate care of a sick woman and involves a well child also. If an elderly person living alone has a minor stroke which limits their independence by making it difficult to cook, clean or shop, another sort of problem arises that might best be solved by a home help, meals on wheels or laundry services. The social worker will help in assessing the need for this service, and in setting up these forms of care if they are needed. Again, if family tensions threaten dangers to the wife or children, supervision and counselling may be required and is most likely to be dealt with by a social worker.

There are some specialised social workers — these include psychiatric social workers who are important in the mechanism that exists for involuntary admission of the psychiatrically sick and in helping and supporting the long term sick such as patients who are schizophrenics, or those with senile dementia who now live in the community.

COMMUNITY PSYCHIATRIC NURSES

Community psychiatric nurses belong to a profession which, although still in its infancy, is of increasing importance. Their role has developed with the trend towards rehabilitating and caring for the mentally infirm in the community. Although they may be based in psychiatric hospitals they are largely involved in providing support and treatment in collaboration with general practitioners. They tend to act as independent clinical practitioners themselves, backed by both consultants and general practitioners, with the object of restricting long-term hospital treatment to the severest cases only.

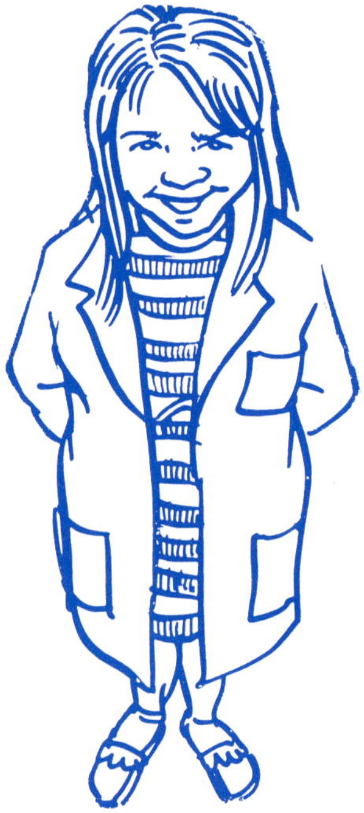

PHARMACISTS

We see in another section how doctors and pharmacists relate to each other in terms of their activities with prescriptions. Many patients go first to the pharmacist with their complaint and may never need to see the doctor. Others are advised by the pharmacist that a consultation is necessary. Communication between the two professions is very important.

HOME HELPS

Home helps play a vital role in keeping the elderly in their homes for as long as possible. Their role is to perform those domestic tasks — such as shopping, washing, cleaning and collecting pensions — which the elderly can no longer undertake because of infirmity. They have no clinical responsibility but their visits provide a friendly and caring link with the outside world. It is usually the Social Services department of the local authority that organises their work.

OTHER MEMBERS

There is a large variety of other skilled workers who, from time to time, become part of the team. Experts like chiropodists, dieticians, physiotherapists, clinical psychologists, pharmacists and so on, may be involved.

The principle skill of the clinical psychologists is in the realm of personal development and interpersonal relationship. They can help with behavioural problems of children and teenagers, getting people to cope with life's difficulties, marital unrest and so on.

HOME CARE TEAMS

We have seen that some teams consist of people employed by the practice, whilst others consist of people employed by the health authorities. There is yet another arm of support — voluntary organisations. A particularly good example of this is the Hospice providing care for the terminally ill. Doctors and nurses working in this field, supported mainly by charity, develop a particular expertise and have teams that can visit patients in their own homes by arrangement with the general practitioner.

The above sections cover the most usual ways in which doctors work with other carers as a team. Local or specialised needs often mean that doctors have to work with agencies or professionals in ways that are not discussed in this chapter.

? Are there other members of the health team in your practice that you could describe?

? How do you communicate with, say, nurses or midwives in your practice?
Is there room for improvement?

? Can you describe a problem associated with working in a team from which your group can learn?

EMERGENCIES

A common source of anxiety to a receptionist is what to do when faced with an emergency. Occasionally this may happen within the surgery when there are no medical or nursing skills available on the premises but most often it is the result of a telephone call. It is valuable if all receptionists learn basic first aid. Topics that should be covered are:

Cardiac and respiratory resuscitation
Care of the unconscious patient
Immediate care of overdose, especially in children
Dealing with haemorrhage
Dealing with suspected fracture

These can usually be covered in one or two evenings and the practice might consider running a refresher course each year. Apart from this there should be a series of 'standing orders' available for emergencies. The general practitioner has a responsibility to provide all necessary care night and day, but clearly cannot personally be available all the time. Anyone who receives messages should have at hand clear instructions about getting quick access to advice or help, and the practice should have a written and agreed policy.

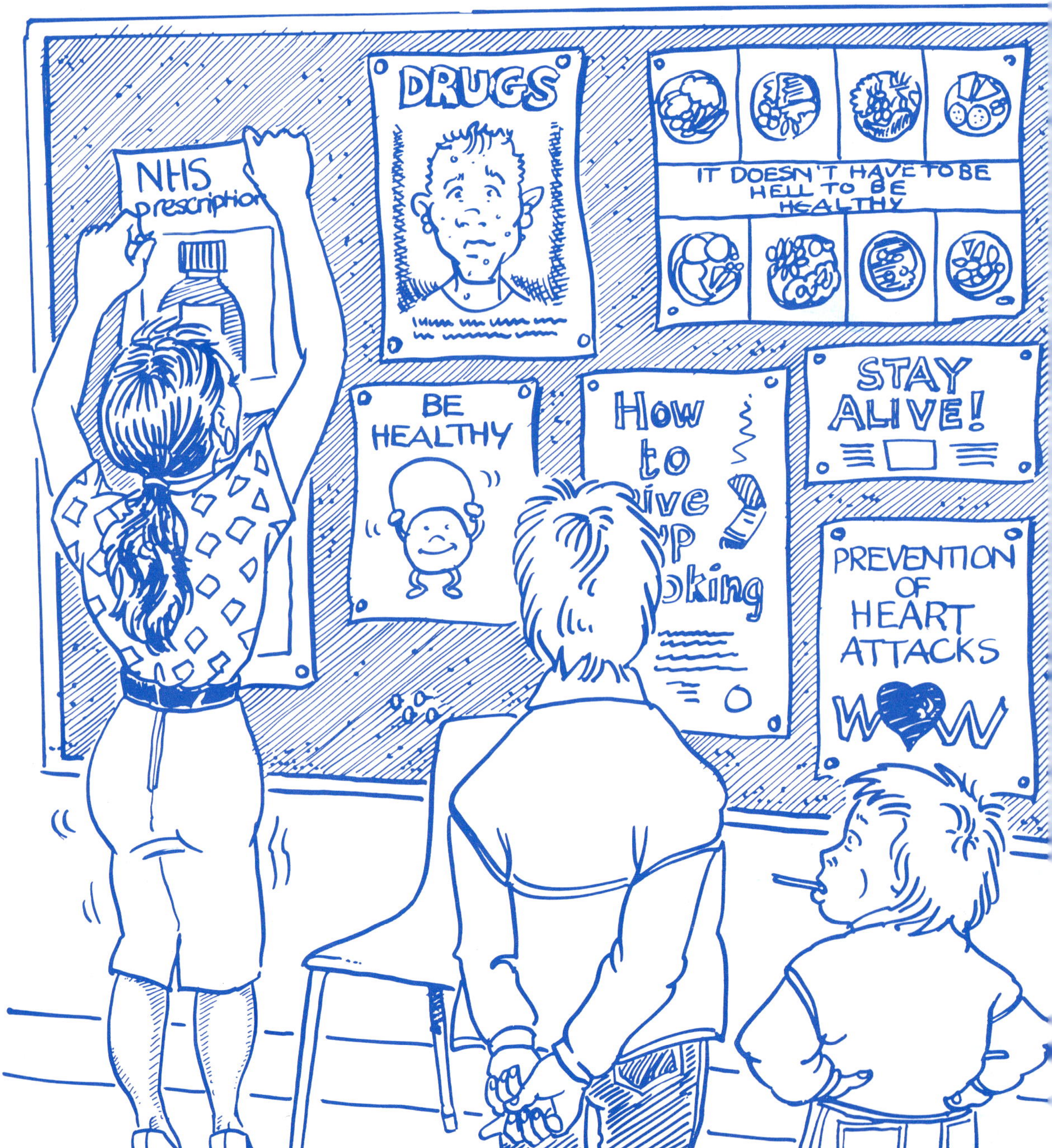
NHS
DRUGS
IT DOESN'T HAVE TO BE HELL TO BE HEALTHY
BE HEALTHY
How to
STAY ALIVE!
PREVENTION OF HEART ATTACKS

7

PREVENTIVE MEDICINE AND HEALTH EDUCATION

In Chapter 9 we shall see how an age/sex register is used to help with preventive care. In this section we shall consider some of the illnesses that we are trying to prevent as this will help show why certain steps are taken. The problems are concerned with high blood pressure, smoking, cervical cancer, excessive alcohol intake, obesity and immunisation against infectious disease.

HIGH BLOOD PRESSURE

Having a sustained blood pressure above normal (hypertension) increases the wear and tear upon the blood vessels and the heart. It is not the only thing that does this, but may increase the effect of other factors such as age, diabetes and smoking, all of which will accelerate the 'furring up' of blood vessels or what is called arterio- or athero-sclerosis.

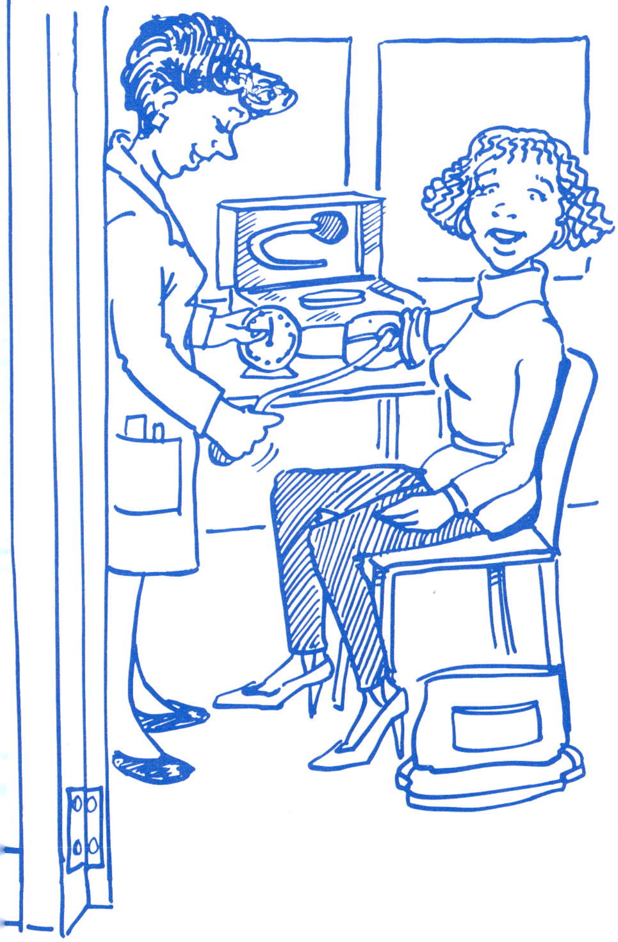

The pressure in blood vessels is not constant and unchanging, but goes up and down according to the time of day, the amount of worry or exercise and so on, so a single reading of the blood pressure does not mean very much. Readings ought to be taken after a person has been sitting quietly for several minutes and is relaxed, and the process should be repeated several times before you can be certain that the pressure is raised.

During the last thirty years a succession of drugs has been discovered that will lower blood pressure and, more significantly, has been shown to reduce the risk of premature stroke or heart failure. These drugs may also lower the numbers of young or middle-aged people who suffer from heart attacks, but this is not certain. Most of these drugs have some unwanted side-effects. The reason why there are so many drugs available is the continuing search for a drug which has the maximum benefit with minimum side-effects. Once the preventive effect of drugs was proven, it became important for us to identify anyone in the population with high blood pressure. The condition only arises in people over the age of thirty to thirty-five years (except for some very rare forms found in the young), so the search has been concentrated amongst the adults over this age. As we are not quite certain how valuable discovering patients over seventy years of age might be — it might be shutting the stable door after the horse has bolted — we usually stop hunting for new cases who are over that age.

At present it seems desirable to divide adults into three groups: those with blood pressure that is normal and below (low blood pressure is not a disease) who need their blood pressures rechecked at intervals of three to five years; those with blood pressures just above normal (mild hypertension) who do not need treatment yet but who should be checked each year; and, those on treatment for hypertension who need to be seen three or four times a year by the nurse or doctor. Raised blood pressure, as we said, is only one factor in causing disease so prevention in practice requires a search for other factors at the same time. Smoking is a major contributor to heart disease and advice must be given to all to stop completely. Excessive alcohol intake and obesity are two other major factors. There are also opportunities at consultation to give general advice on diet and exercise, although it is not certain that these contribute excessively to causing high blood pressure.

SMOKING

The link between smoking and cancer of the bronchus was discovered more than twenty years ago. It is one of the most proven links between any cause and a cancer, but in spite of this many people continue to smoke, even after they have received treatment for the disease. Smoking is also related to other cancers and diseases and it has been estimated that the number of deaths from smoking related diseases in the United Kingdom would only be equalled by having three fully laden jumbo jets crashing every week.

Smoking rates have declined fastest amongst higher social class males and slowest amongst lower social class females. The death rates have dropped proportionately in these groups. In fact amongst women it is still rising due to the increased number of women who started smoking twenty to thirty years ago. The risk is greater with the increased number of cigarettes smoked and gets lower as soon as smoking is stopped, returning to normal about ten years after stopping smoking. It is particularly dangerous for expectant mothers who have been shown to have a higher rate of miscarriage and smaller babies than non-smoking mothers. It appears to be harmful to those who live or work with smokers, or in smoky atmospheres, even if they do not smoke themselves.

There have been many studies directed at trying to find the most effective source of advice for patients about smoking. Several of these studies have shown that general practice is the best place. Advice and help on how to stop smoking has become part of normal consulting activity. Other people, such as clinical psychologists, are of value and other methods such as chewing gum containing nicotine or the use of hypnosis may help, but whatever method is used it requires the efforts of all in health care to lower the toll of unnecessary death and suffering.

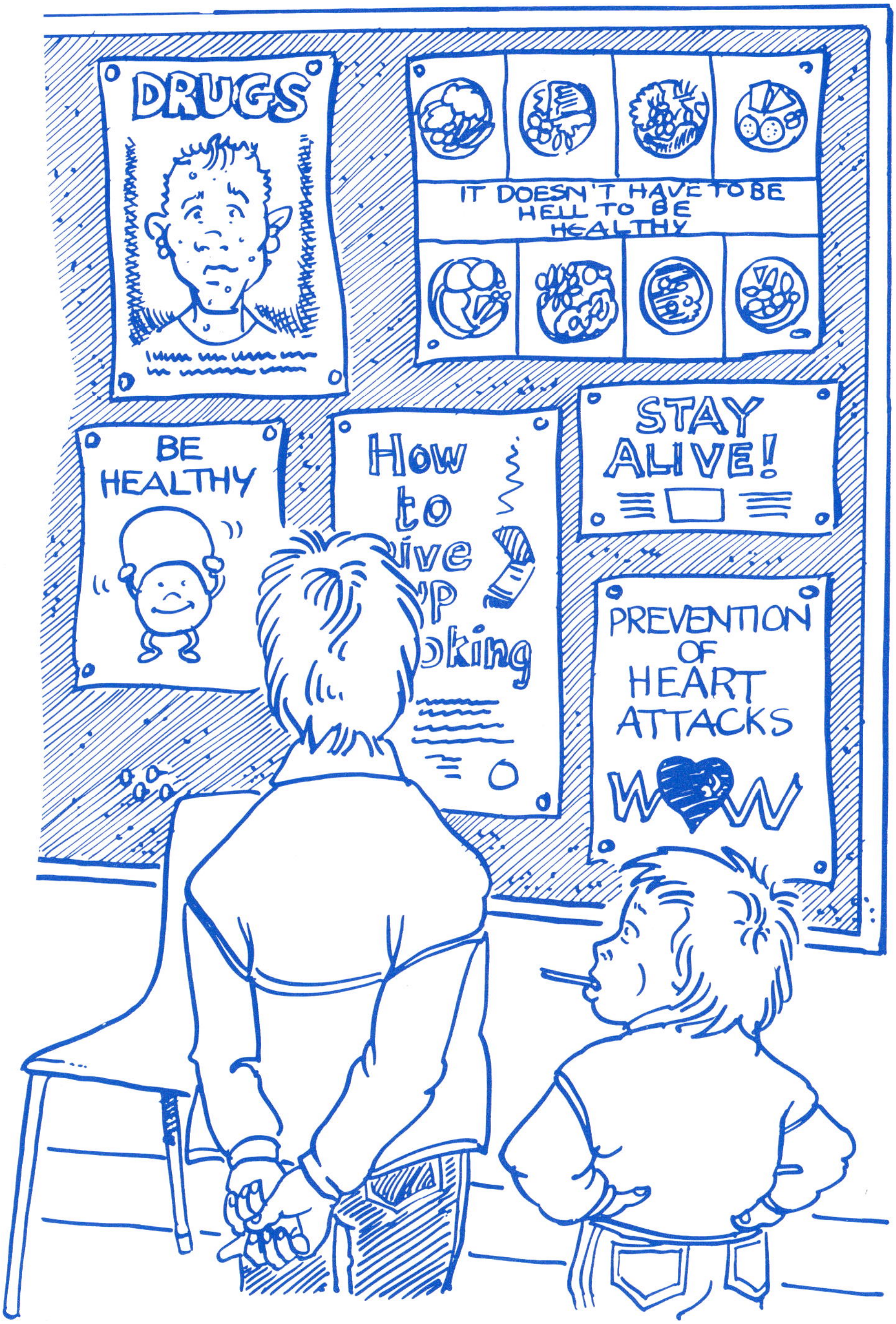

CERVICAL CANCER

The cause of cervical cancer is unknown but various theories suggest a viral infection of the cells on the cervix. Untreated, cervical cancer will eventually cause death, which in younger women may be quite rapid. Some of the factors associated with the development of this cancer have been identified and behavioural changes may lower the incidence. For example, it does seem to be associated with early sexual experience and with the number of sexual partners. We also know that there is a latent period, which might be quite long, between developing some changes in the cervical cell and developing cancer, and that a relatively simple form of treatment in the intervening period can prevent it developing; hence the cervical smear and subsequent treatment.

There is now a widespread campaign to persuade women to have regular smears, starting soon after they have become sexually active and continuing until they are over sixty years old. This campaign makes use of case finding and screening. Patients may have smears in hospital, in family planning clinics or in the surgery. The results normally return to the practice, wherever the smear was carried out, and as the G.P's record is the only continuous and comprehensive health record relating to the patient it is vital that results go into the record and are clearly identifiable.

We shall see in other sections how the age/sex register, the follow up system and the records themselves form an inter-relating system in preventive care.

EXCESSIVE ALCOHOL INTAKE

Men should not drink more than twenty-one units of alcohol a week, and women not more than fourteen units. For both men and women this should include two or three days each week without any alcohol. One unit is a single measure of spirit or one glass of wine or sherry or half a pint of beer. The amount of alcohol consumed is increasing and we now spend more on this than we do on clothes, cars, hospitals or education. It has been estimated that in a practice of 2,000 patients, 135 would be heavy drinkers, forty problem drinkers — that is their work or life is affected by drinking — and seven would be alcohol-dependent patients.

It is not certain how much disease is caused by overdrinking but it is substantial and it is becoming more common for general practitioners to enquire into the drinking habits of patients and to add advice. It is certainly a factor in causing high blood pressure, cancer of various organs, liver damage and disease, as well as marital breakup, stress on children, increased accidents and crimes of violence.

OBESITY

It is unlikely that weight causes disease until it is more than twenty-five per cent above normal. At lower levels it causes fatigue, shortness of breath and discomfort. It is an aggravating feature in some diseases such as arthritis of the hips and knees and hiatus hernia. Doctors are sometimes effective at helping patients to lose weight when they are able to demonstrate that symptoms can be improved by losing weight. At other times practice nurses can help, and organisations such as 'weight-watchers' are useful.

IMMUNISATION AGAINST INFECTIOUS DISEASE

The range of diseases that can be prevented by immunisation is increasing. Immunisation depends upon the principle that sometimes the administration of a dead organism, or one that has been treated to make it relatively harmless, can stimulate the person so treated to produce antibodies to the organism which will protect that person should he or she later come into contact with it.

We immunise children against polio, diphtheria, tetanus, whooping cough (pertussis) and tuberculosis. We also use measles and mumps vaccines and shortly a combined vaccine against measles, mumps and rubella will be available. In healthy adults we try to keep the immune levels against polio and tetanus at high levels and we use vaccines to protect individuals at risk (those dealing with, or coming into contact with, human blood) against hepatitis. We immunise teenage girls against german measles (rubella), and also women of child-bearing age. Finally we try to protect travellers going overseas against diseases endemic in the countries to be visited.

Diphtheria killed more than 2,500 people in the U.K. (mainly children) in 1941 but now there are virtually no deaths from this disease. Its absence depends upon keeping a high level of immunisation in the community.

Tetanus causes a few deaths every year. It can be completely prevented by immunisation and everyone — receptionists as well — should be immunised and have a booster at five to ten year intervals. Tetanus is particularly associated with severe and dirty wounds but can occur even after an event as minor as a prick by a rosethorn, since the spores lie dormant in the soil for many years.

Tuberculosis is a worldwide problem, but its incidence in developed countries has fallen because of better social conditions and vaccination. It still causes several hundred deaths each year in the U.K. and has a higher incidence amongst Asian immigrants. The disease is caused by one of two forms of a bacillus, the human form, which most often causes chest disease, and the bovine or cattle form, which is in most cases associated with glandular infection. The initial infection usually heals without causing illness but confers some immunity and converts skin tests (Mantoux, Heaf) to positive. Skin testing is performed in this country on children aged ten to thirteen years and is organised at school. For those who are negative (who have not had a first or primary infection) an intradermal injection of B.C.G. (Bacille Calmette Guerin), which is a weakened form of the cattle organism, is given.

A mumps vaccine is now being widely introduced. Its importance lies in its ability to prevent mumps in adults, where serious complications involving testes or ovaries can cause infertility, and where other glands such as the pancreas may be affected.

Hepatitis comes in two forms, hepatitis A and hepatitis B. Type A is caused by a virus and is spread in contaminated food or water. It is a nasty illness but not usually dangerous. Type B virus is very different. About one in a hundred sufferers from it die and ten in a hundred get chronic liver disease. It is usually spread by an injection of blood or blood products so drug users and people who work with syringes and needles such as doctors, dentists and nurses are most at risk.

Whooping cough (pertussis) immunisation has been surrounded by controversy linked with its dangers but there is no doubt at all that the risks, to life and health, of whooping cough greatly outweigh any risks from the vaccine. It is particularly dangerous in infancy.

Measles occurs in epidemics every other year. It is spread by children whose very early symptoms may appear to be those of just a bad cold. Common complications of measles are ear infections and chest infections. More rare are infections of the brain.

Poliomyelitis disappeared from Britain due to the immunisation programme in the 1970's. It affects children and young adults mainly causing paralysis of muscles which may never recover. It is important to maintain the immune levels of adults under 40 years of age by a reinforcing dose especially those who are travelling to Third World countries.

Rubella is a minor illness in children. In pregnancy however it may cause deafness, blindness or heart disease in the foetus and we attempt to produce immunity in all females before they are at child-bearing age.

FOREIGN TRAVEL

The diseases commonly protected against include typhoid fever, which requires a first course of two injections and booster doses every two years, and cholera in which immunity conferred by immunisation only lasts for three to six months.

Yellow fever and hepatitis immunisation and protection against hepatitis are less commonly required but they are life threatening diseases so in some areas of the world protection is vital. Malaria prophylaxis is strongly indicated for travellers. There are now, unfortunately, many resistant organisms and the exact requirements for each area are specified by experts. Tablets need to be taken before travel and continued for six weeks after leaving the infectious area. One of the biggest problems of foreign travel is AIDS for which no vaccine is available but prevention is essential.

In this section on preventive medicine we have considered some of the more obvious ways in which ill health can be prevented. In fact every consultation with a doctor, nurse or receptionist may provide an opportunity to practise preventive care. You may wish to discuss how this can be done by receptionists.

? What role do you have in supporting preventive measures in your practice?

? What sources of information about immunisation and prevention of disease are available in your surgery?

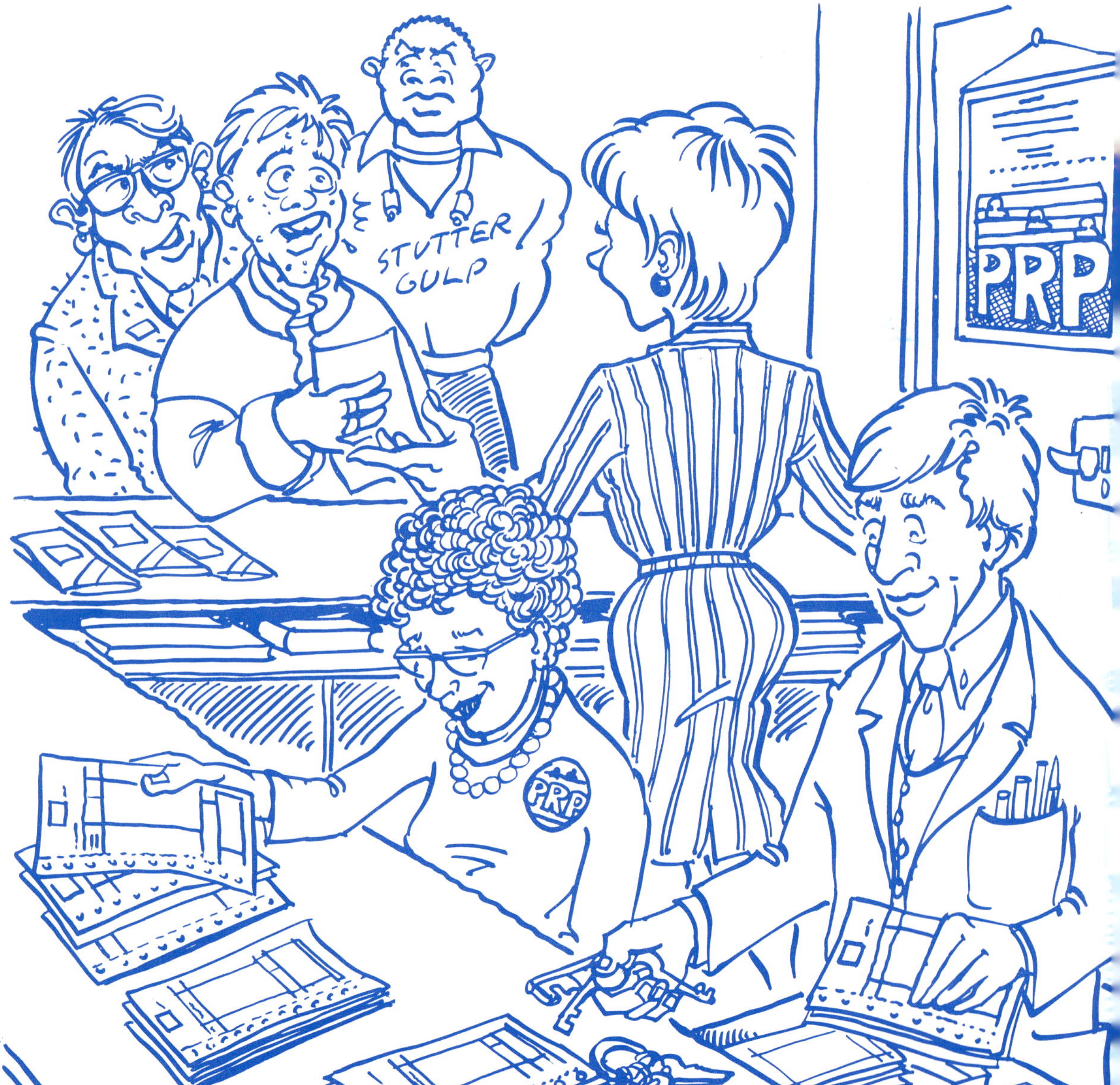
STUTTER
GULP
PRP
PRP

8

PRESCRIPTIONS AND THE RECEPTIONIST

General practitioners in Britain write more than 400 million prescriptions every year. In 1986 each prescription contained, on average, over £5 worth of drugs so the total cost was over £2,000,000,000. The great majority of these were for National Health patients and were written on forms FP10 (GP10 Scot). Prescribing is not something that the doctor does at every consultation and even when he does it is not always the most important part of treatment — reassurance and advice often come first. Of all the prescriptions written, only about half are given to the patient by the doctor. In all the others the receptionist will be involved either in receiving the request for the prescription and in handing it out (or posting it) to the patient, or in writing all or part of the prescription. In every practice several hours every day are occupied with these prescriptions. This activity has become so important that it deserves a chapter to itself.

The doctor has ultimate responsibility for all prescribing issued under his or her name. It is of paramount importance that practice procedures, including those covering the issue of prescriptions, both originals and repeats, are agreed with the doctor. Preferably procedures should be recorded for reference purposes to ensure that everyone working in the practice is familiar with them and understands their particular responsibility. A procedure should establish safe and efficient methods which reflect current good standards of practice. Checking procedures should be built into all the systems operated in a practice and are especially important where prescriptions are concerned.

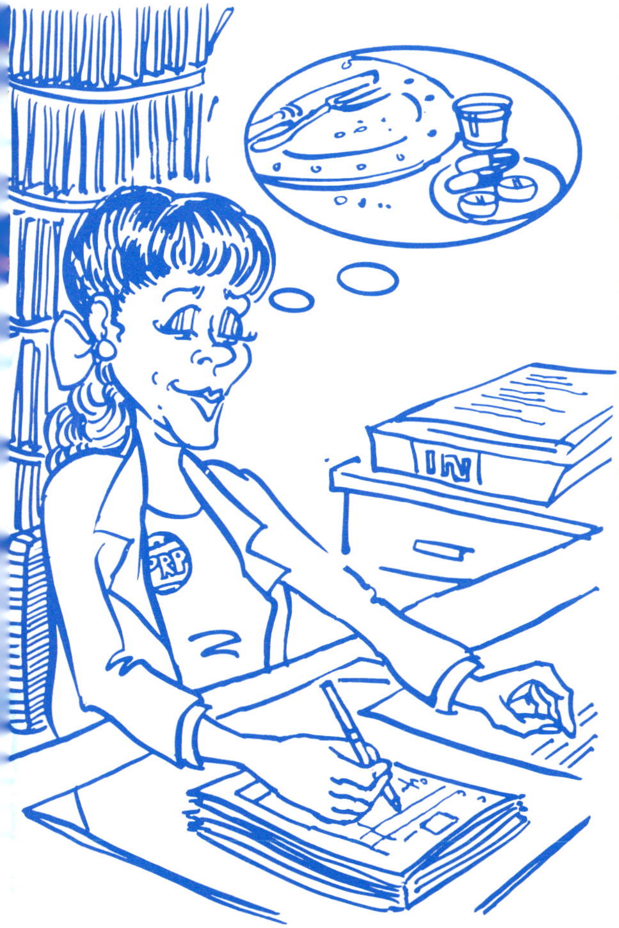

WRITING A PRESCRIPTION

A prescription is a request to a pharmacist to supply medicine. Normally a prescription will contain several sections:

A The full identification details of the patient. These must be written legibly in ink or typewritten and should contain the patient's title (Mr, Mrs or Miss), surname, initials and one full forename. These details will be put on the container by the pharmacist and this will help to make sure that the right medicine gets to the right patient. Form FP10 (GP10 Scot) has a box at the top for the age of children under twelve. This must be completed as an additional check that an adult dose is not given to a child.

B The name of the medicine/s to be dispensed. This must be written very clearly. Many drugs have very similar names, for example hydralazine and hydrenox, or chlorpropamide and chlorpromazine. A twelve-year-old child died as a result of getting the wrong drug when a pharmacist misread the poor writing on a prescription for the latter. A coroner recorded a verdict of death by misadventure. Most drugs have two names, a proprietary or trade name given to them by the manufacturer and a generic or approved name given when the drug is licensed for sale. This is a bit confusing but we often use this device in other fields. For example 'petrol' is a generic name and 'Esso' or 'B.P.' are proprietary brands. There is debate as to whether prescribing by generic name should be encouraged or not. The medicines are usually cheaper when provided by generic names, and these names indicate the chemical family to which the drug belongs, which may help the doctor, for example diazepam, lorazepam, nitrazepam and lormetazepam are all from the same 'family'. Unfortunately the names are usually longer and more difficult to spell! Most doctors try to prescribe by generic name when they can but it is sometimes confusing for the patient if at times they have a generic drug supplied quite correctly under one proprietary name and at other times under a different proprietary name especially when the two varieties may look quite different. They can however be reassured that the medicine is just the same and just as safe and effective. The name of the drug, as indicated on the prescription, will be put on the label by the pharmacist unless the doctor has put a cross in the box labelled NP at the top of form FP10 to indicate to the pharmacist not to do so.

C The dose of the drug. For solids this is given in grams (g) or milligrams (mg). If a decimal point is used a zero should be added first (0·25 mg). For liquids the dose is given in millilitres (ml). Micrograms must always be written in full.

D The frequency of doses to be taken, for example 'three times a day' or 'at night'. There is still a tendency to use abbreviations of English or Latin phrases but they should now be avoided, so it is better to write 'at night' rather than 'o.n.' (omni nocte).

E The quantity to be supplied. When possible it is a good idea to use the box on form FP10 to indicate the number of days of treatment. The pharmacist will then work out the number of tablets required. This is a particular help if the patient is taking several medicines, some once a day, some twice and some three times, as they will all last the patient the same length of time. Sometimes when a preparation is supplied prepacked in a fixed quantity, such as an ointment that is only available in a 30 g tube it will suffice to put 'original pack' or O.P. as an indication of the quantity, but it is best to be specific.

F Other instructions such as 'before meals' or 'with water' will be added but the pharmacist may add these instructions by following recommended guidelines contained in the British National Formulary, without this being on the prescription.

The drugs with which a doctor is mainly concerned come into the category of 'prescription only medicines' (P.O.M.). They can only be issued by a practitioner and have to be signed by the doctor though, of course, dentists and vets have their own range of drugs under this category that they may prescribe. The following rules governing prescription of these medicines are laid down in Acts of Parliament and Regulations and they must be obeyed:

1 All prescriptions have to be signed by the doctor and the prescription must contain his name, address and the date.

2 Controlled drugs must contain certain particulars in the prescribing doctor's own handwriting. These are the patient's own name and address, all the details of the drug and the amount written in figures and words. This means that the receptionist cannot make out any part of these prescriptions. It is essential that prescriptions for controlled drug items should be complete in all respects in order to avoid problems when the prescriptions are presented for dispensing. These rules apply to private prescriptions as well as those written on National Health Service forms.

'Controlled' drugs are those such as morphine and heroin which have the potential to cause addiction or other harmful side-effects.

3 In addition it will be necessary to comply with the requirements of the 'Limited List'. Drugs not on this list are excluded from N.H.S. prescribing on the grounds of economy and alleged lack of proven effectiveness; doctors can still prescribe them however, but only on a private prescription.

SECURITY

Prescriptions are of course valuable documents. They are important to the patient who wants to get his medicine accurately and promptly prescribed but they have also unfortunately become important to others as well. The commonest reason the doctor's surgery is broken into is to steal drugs, but blank prescription forms that can later be forged or sold are equally valuable. At the end of every day prescription pads must be locked away.

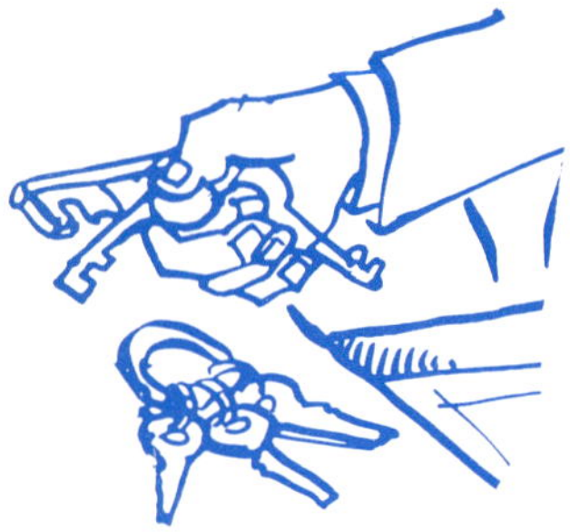

Those on the doctor's desk should be locked in a drawer in the desk and the supply of spare forms kept in as burglar-proof a place as possible. Finally, any prescriptions that are made out for controlled drugs (a list of special drugs that are liable to be misused by some people) should be kept in a secure place until they are handed over to the patient. Under no circumstances should presigned, blank prescriptions ever be available in the practice. Theft of FP10 (GP10 Scot) forms should be reported to the F.P.C. immediately, thereafter the prescribing doctor will be issued with a pad of forms bearing details of the doctor's name and address printed in red. Local pharmacies will be alerted to the theft and to the issue of the special forms. Subsequent telephone calls from a pharmacist suspecting a forged prescription should be dealt with urgently.

REPEAT PRESCRIBING

As nearly half of all the prescriptions issued are repeats — that is they are made out without a consultation taking place at that time — they may take up a considerable part of the receptionist's working day. There are many different ways of dealing with them but it should be remembered that the easiest system for practice staff is not necessarily the most appropriate system for patient safety. Some practices have stopped issuing repeat prescriptions altogether and this seems to work for them. Other practices use repeat prescription cards for some or all of these scripts and an increasing number have them produced by microcomputer — so it is not possible to recommend a 'best buy'. There are however some important general rules that you can identify in discussion within your groups. You can then see whether all or some of these can be made to apply to your practice. They are concerned with such notions as availability, reliability, records and follow-up. You may want to ask and answer questions under these headings.

There should be clear indications within the practice as to which patients are 'eligible' for repeat prescriptions.

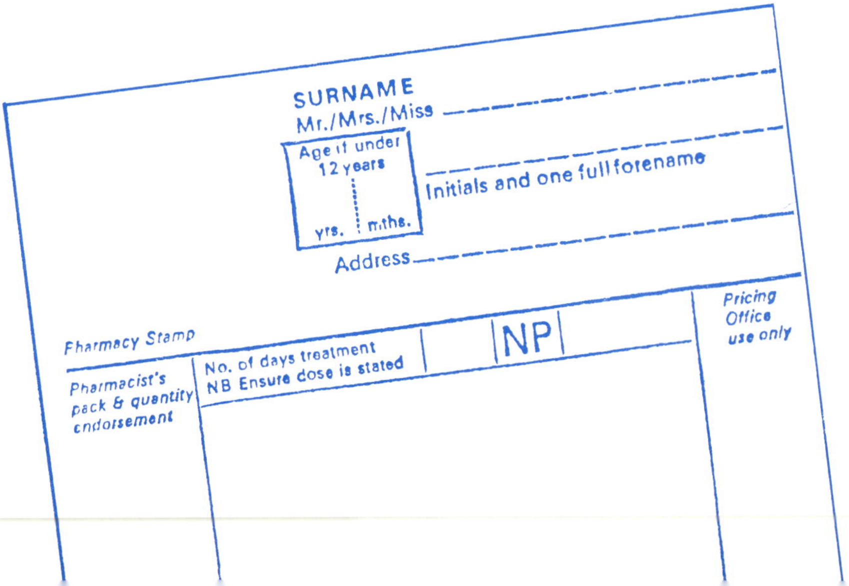

How can patients request and receive their prescriptions most easily?

How do you make it easy for them to identify which drugs they want?

How do you make it easier for them to collect their scripts? Do you post them? Do you ever forward them to a pharmacy identified by the patient?

How can it be made easier for you to prepare their prescription?

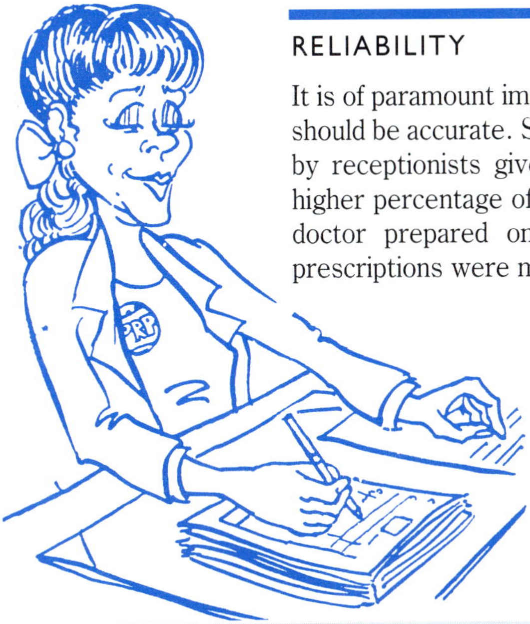

RELIABILITY

It is of paramount importance that the details recorded on the prescription should be accurate. Studies that have been done on prescriptions prepared by receptionists give contradictory results. One showed there to be a higher percentage of errors in receptionist prepared prescriptions than in doctor prepared ones, but other studies showed that receptionists' prescriptions were more legible than doctors'.

What documents might you need to refer to when preparing a prescription?

What information might you find in them?

What do you want to find in the records when writing repeat prescriptions?

How do you deal with repeat prescription cards?

What methods of checking accuracy do you operate (including self checking)?

What are the advantages and the disadvantages?

RECORDS

It might be agreed that any system should enable a receptionist to prepare a prescription (other than for a controlled drug) on behalf of the prescriber and enter it in the patient's records.

? Are your patient records maintained on a computer?

Can it be used to prepare prescriptions?

? What problems have there been and how have they been overcome?

? How do you operate a repeat prescription system in your practice?

? How do you keep them up-to-date?

What record is made in the notes?

? How are the patients for whom repeat prescriptions may be issued identified in your records (manual or computer)?

FOLLOW-UP

The increase in the number of repeat prescriptions over the last few years is said to be mainly due to the rise in the importance given to the care of chronic disease in the general practitioner's work and to the availability of modern drug treatment. The number of consultations required for good care of patients suffering from hypertension, diabetes, asthma, arthritis and angina is increasing, partly because we now have more effective drugs, partly because there is a gradual shift from hospital to community care, and partly because we now know that good control will stop the development of complications and improve the quality of life. Many of these patients will need to see the doctor or nurse relatively infrequently and probably less frequently than they need a prescription refilled. These requests for repeat prescriptions can be used as a 'trigger' mechanism for recall and for monitoring progress.

What sort of recall system do you use for monitoring patients on repeat prescriptions?

How can you check on a patient's compliance?

How do you look out for patient abuse of your repeat prescription system?

There are a number of other areas in relation to prescribing that we have not covered. Private prescriptions may have to be written either for private patients, for patients who are going abroad, or for substances that are not available on the N.H.S., such as certain foodstuffs or cosmetics. Doctors will have to keep in the surgery stocks of drugs to be given by injection or substances for diagnostic purposes.

When problems arise in prescribing for patients, close communication is required between the doctor and the pharmacist. Whenever the pharmacist has difficulty in dispensing because of an error in the prescription or because, say, a preparation is not available, he will ask the patient to take the prescription back to the doctor or, more commonly, will telephone the doctor. The pharmacist is an extremely important source of information and the relationship between the medical and the pharmaceutical professions must be close.

9

AGE/SEX REGISTER

One of the most significant changes that has taken place in general practice in the past twenty years has been the gradual shift from 'reacting' to a problem to trying to 'prevent' it arising. This involves a change in attitude amongst doctors and staff and a change in organisation within the practice. These changes have not yet been made by everyone, but they will. Put most simply they can be expressed as a different requirement of the patient who is 'signing on' with the doctor. Ten years ago they might have been assumed to have been asking questions such as 'Will you come to see me if I have a pain or if I break my leg?' To that is now added an implied question 'and will you stop my family catching polio, or getting cancer of the cervix or suffering from a stroke whilst young?' To be efficient in this latter task takes a very big attitudinal change and a very considerable addition to the organisation.

It is, perhaps, important to put some cautionary words in at this point. Not everything can be prevented, and even where it can it is important that the benefits from doing so are balanced against the cost. It may just be too expensive to take on some medical tasks if that means that others of more potential benefit have to be left undone. Working out priorities in medicine is often very difficult. Another cautionary word relates to the freedom of the individual. The patient should always be at liberty to say 'No'; to say that they do not want this investigation or that injection to be performed. The refusal should however be an informed one. That is to say the patient's decision must be based on good information and not on ignorance. It therefore implies that the surgery staff have a responsibility to ensure that patients and their families understand the need for preventive measures.

In another section of this book we consider what can be prevented and how, and the benefits of using computers in record-keeping. In this section we shall think about the systems required to practise preventive care.

The most important feature of primary care within the National Health Service is the existence of a list of individual patients registered with one doctor. This means that every item of care applied to that patient anywhere in the health service is eventually recorded in that patient's notes. It is therefore possible that every time the patient has an item of preventive care, such as the recording of a blood pressure or an immunisation against tetanus, it will be recorded in the general practice notes and will become that patient's notes for life. Because all the patients' notes on the doctor's list will be in the files it will be possible to scrutinise them to find out, for instance, who has had their blood pressure recorded in the previous five years and, more importantly, who has not. Steps could then be taken to contact the patients without blood pressure recordings so that almost a hundred per cent of people at risk could be dealt with. In fact in most practices studies show figures of only seventy per cent immunised against infectious disease, sixty per cent of at risk women who have had cervical smears, and fifty per cent of adult men with a recent blood pressure recording. There are two methods of improving on these figures; screening and case finding.

Screening consists of sending for the 'at risk' population. For example a letter could be sent to all women aged between thirty-five years and sixty-five years inviting them to attend the surgery. In some practices this has been shown to work quite well but is relatively expensive. For an average practice of say 10,000 people it would involve about 2,000 women, which means sending 2,000 letters, stamps and replies, and having a system to cope with the 1,200 estimated replies, as well as the estimated 800 who do not reply. This procedure might have to be repeated for a number of different conditions within the same population. Some practices get round this problem by inviting 'well people' to attend the same consultation for a series of different procedures: there are 'well baby clinics', 'well women clinics' and 'well men clinics'. These people may be sent for or there may be a walk-in system with or without an appointment. All of these systems come under the category of screening.

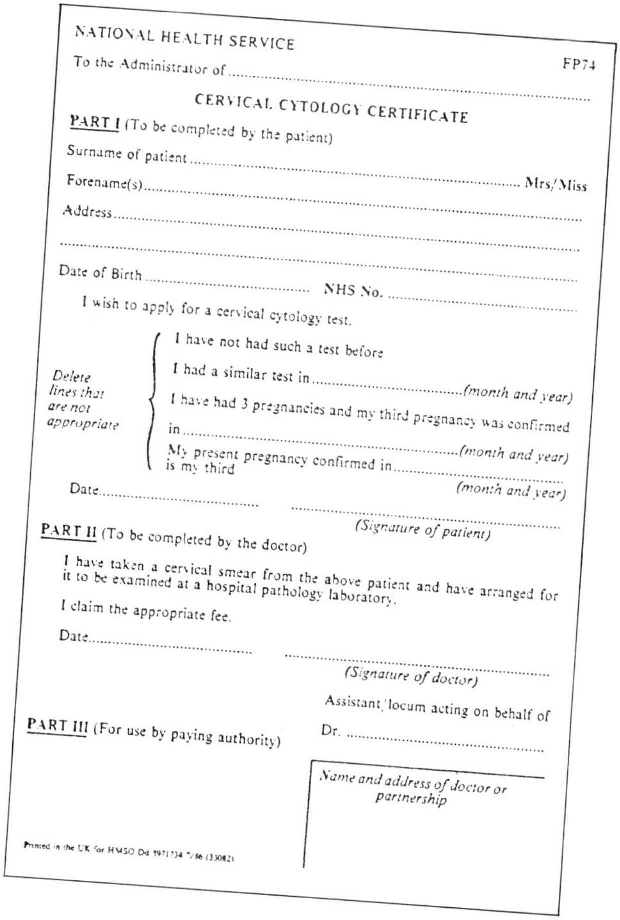

NATIONAL HEALTH SERVICE

To the Administrator of FP74

CERVICAL CYTOLOGY CERTIFICATE

PART I (To be completed by the patient)

Surname of patient ....

Forename(s) .... Mrs/Miss

Address ....

....

Date of Birth .... NHS No. ....

I wish to apply for a cervical cytology test.

Delete lines that are not appropriate
- I have not had such a test before
- I had a similar test in .... *(month and year)*
- I have had 3 pregnancies and my third pregnancy was confirmed in .... *(month and year)*
- My present pregnancy confirmed in .... is my third *(month and year)*

Date .... *(Signature of patient)*

PART II (To be completed by the doctor)

I have taken a cervical smear from the above patient and have arranged for it to be examined at a hospital pathology laboratory.

I claim the appropriate fee.

Date .... *(Signature of doctor)*

Assistant/locum acting on behalf of

PART III (For use by paying authority)

Dr. ....

Name and address of doctor or partnership

Printed in the UK for HMSO Dd 1971734 7/86 (33082)

Case finding is quite different. It depends on the principle that in any year about seventy per cent of the practice population will attend the doctor's surgery for one reason or another. When they do attend they can be 'caught' for another purpose, such as taking (or making an appointment for) a cervical smear. Furthermore, by the time two years are up the proportion of attenders will have risen to eighty per cent and to ninety per cent by the end of three years so that only ten per cent will remain to be contacted in some other way. Such a system requires all the surgery staff to be convinced of its importance and to be particularly assiduous in carrying it out.

Clearly it would be a tedious business to scan the records to ascertain the preventive status of the whole practice so a tool called an age/sex register has been devised. This is used in a variety of tasks including research, but it is in preventive medicine that it really comes into its own. The names of all the patients are divided up according to date of birth, and then again by sex. This register may be kept in a book but more frequently a card is made out for each patient. There will be, say, sixty-eight cards filed under 1936 representing all the females aged fifty-two, it is then possible to tag these cards with other information so that the card for Ann Smith, born in 1936, will show that she had a cervical smear in 1986 and

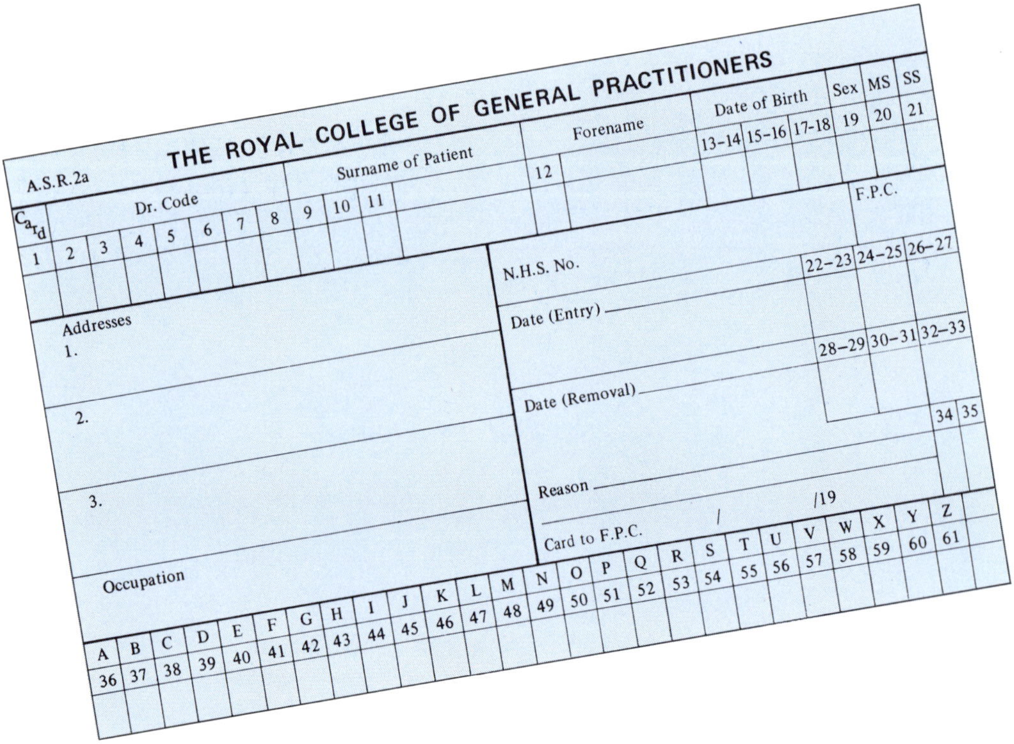

that her blood pressure was checked at the same time. This does not mean that the records for that patient will not have that information in them as well. It will be necessary to seek there for further details and it will also be necessary to use these notes every time a patient attends to 'case find' for other preventive measures that might be needed. When she attends in 1991 with her bunion it will be necessary to check her blood pressure again.

An age/sex register is only as good as the accuracy of the details that it contains so it will require constant maintenance to correct changes of address or name, as well as insertion of the preventive procedures as they are done. At this point you may wish to consider several questions, for example:

Does your practice have policies for dealing with
- cervical smears?
- blood pressures?
- immunisations?

How are these policies decided and communicated?

What staff are involved in this work and what do they do?

What documentation is used in your practice to record the preventive procedures carried out?

Is there an age/sex register in your practice?

How is it kept up-to-date?

What other ways can staff be involved in preventive care?

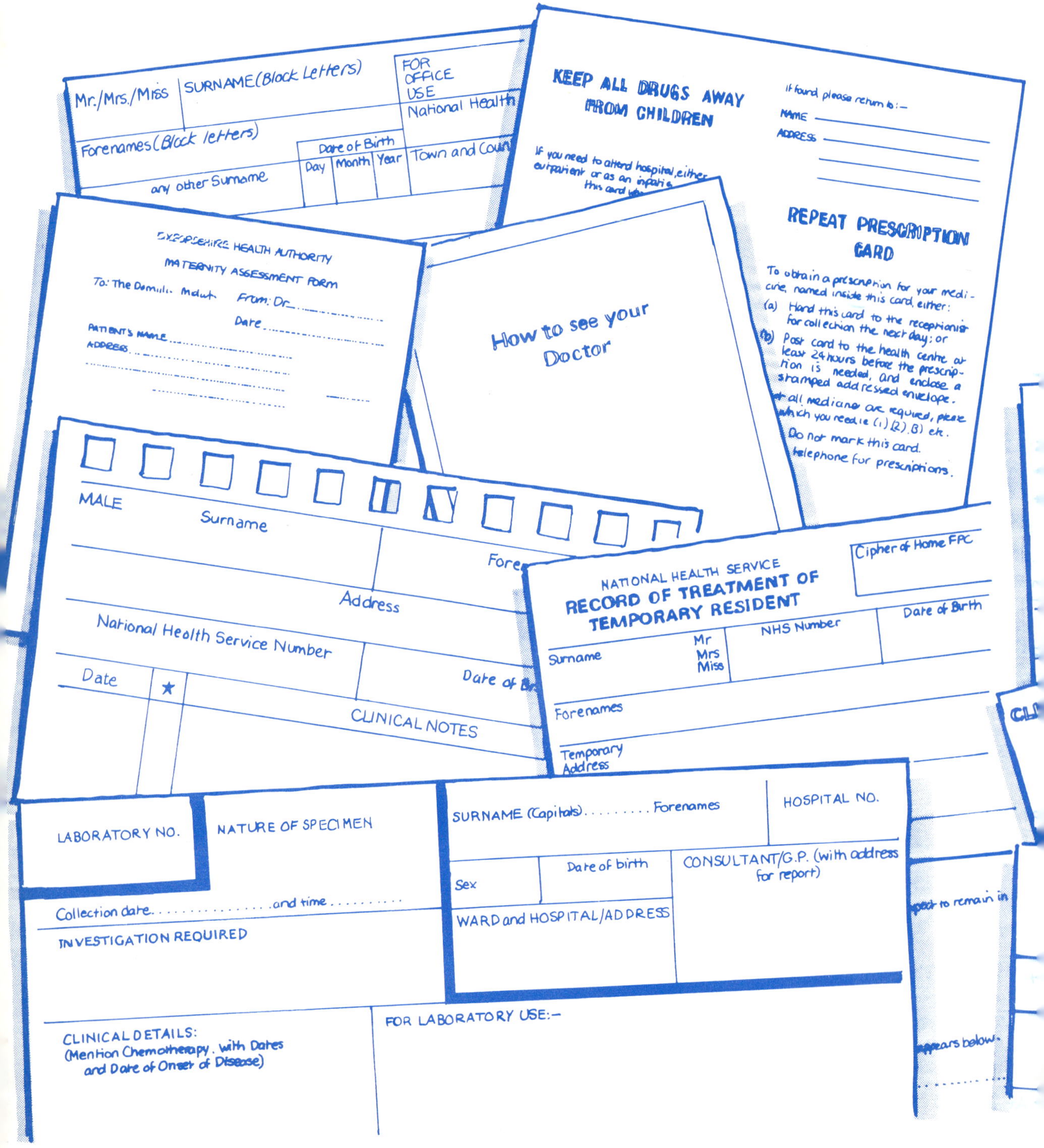
Mr./Mrs./Miss
SURNAME (Block Letters)
FOR OFFICE USE
National Health
Forenames (Block letters)
Date of Birth
Day
Month
Year
Town and Coun
any other Surname
KEEP ALL DRUGS AWAY FROM CHILDREN
If found please return to:-
NAME
ADDRESS
If you need to attend hospital, either outpatient or as an inpatie
this card
REPEAT PRESCRIPTION CARD
To obtain a prescription for your medicine, named inside this card, either:
(a) Hand this card to the receptionist for collection the next day; or
(b) Post card to the health centre at least 24 hours before the prescription is needed, and enclose a stamped addressed envelope.
all medicine are required, please which you need i.e. (1) (2) (3) etc.
Do not mark this card.
telephone for prescriptions.
HEALTH AUTHORITY
MATERNITY ASSESSMENT FORM
To: The Domicili. Midwif.
From: Dr.
Date
PATIENT'S NAME
ADDRESS
How to see your Doctor
MALE
Surname
Fore
Address
National Health Service Number
Date
★
Date of B
CLINICAL NOTES
NATIONAL HEALTH SERVICE
RECORD OF TREATMENT OF TEMPORARY RESIDENT
Cipher of Home FPC
Date of Birth
NHS Number
Surname
Mr
Mrs
Miss
Forenames
Temporary Address
LABORATORY NO.
NATURE OF SPECIMEN
Collection date.................and time..........
INVESTIGATION REQUIRED
CLINICAL DETAILS:
(Mention Chemotherapy. with Dates and Date of Onset of Disease)
FOR LABORATORY USE:-
SURNAME (Capitals).........Forenames
HOSPITAL NO.
Sex
Date of birth
CONSULTANT/G.P. (with address for report)
WARD and HOSPITAL/ADDRESS
pect to remain in
appears below.

10 RECORDS AND FORMS

It was said by one cynic that a doctor could work perfectly well today without a stethoscope but if he had not got his pen with him he was immobilised. Whilst this is obviously an exaggeration it does have a grain of truth concealed within it, for medical records are an essential part of care, and without them good care is quite impossible. General practice is handicapped to some extent by having to rely on medical records that were designed over seventy years ago. It is said that the standard 'Lloyd George' envelope was made the shape and size it is so that it could be kept in the surplus ammunition boxes that were left over after the First World War. They may have been adequate in the 1920's when the notes could not be expected to contain more than a diagnosis such as 'neurasthenia' and the words 'Mist. Pot. Brom.' signifying that a bromide mixture had been dispensed (some of these can still be found in the filing cabinets) but it is hardly appropriate for the sophisticated records required today. A small number of practices have converted to A4 size records (hospital note size) and an even smaller number keep their records entirely on computer, but the vast majority still use the old 'Lloyd George' N.H.S. envelopes called FP 5 & 6 (in Scotland GP 5 & 6).

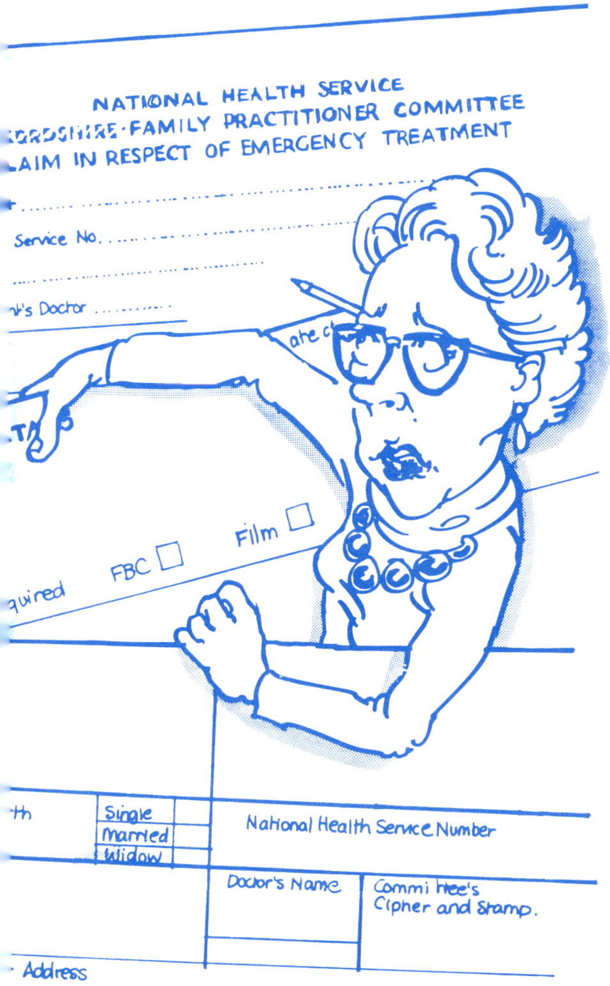

Whilst the contents of the records are the responsibility of the doctor, and the management systems are the prerogative of the practice manager, they are constantly being handled by the receptionist and there are general rules that apply to them.

1 Availability. The importance of the record for patient management has already been stressed. Whenever the doctor is dealing with a patient he must have the records available, for reference, and to enter new details. It may not always be necessary to do this but the more accessible the records, the more meticulous people will be in their recording. Whenever the patient is seen in the surgery or at home, or a telephone conversation is held, or a letter or report is received about the patient, the records should be available. Different practices will have different ways of dealing with this. Some attach incoming reports and letters to the outside of the medical record so that the doctor can see both together. Some receptionists connect the patient's telephone call to the doctor after obtaining his consent and then discreetly arrive with the records so that he can refer to them. Sometimes there is more than one patient with the same surname and forename. It may not be possible to identify the patient involved, so the receptionist might then present the doctor with the records of all three 'Ann Smiths' so that he can be certain of having the right one if needed.

2 Filing. Any records that are not in use should be refiled at the earliest possible moment. Filing is not done to tidy up the office, it is designed to make it easy to retrieve notes. Unfortunately records have a life of their own, and an ability to wander about. They stay for days on people's desks, or in the back of the doctor's car, and no-one knows better than the receptionist how much trouble this causes. Staff all have to be equally disciplined and have to attend to matters promptly so that they can be refiled.

Filing is a skill, some people are accurate and quick at it whilst others have difficulty. There are a number of methods that people use to make the task easier; most people use a tracer card which goes into the file from which the note has been removed; sometimes this is matched with a card that is inserted in the record. Occasionally tracer cards are numbered or of different colours to make the processing quicker. If the records are missing a search has to be made of every room and if they cannot be found quickly a temporary card with the patient's name and number is made out and marked in bold letters 'temporary'. Where files are kept on open shelving some practices mark the spine with a coloured sticker in an organised way so that a misfiled record can be spotted easily. Refiling can be a back-breaking task and an attempt should be made to keep records at a reasonable number and height.

3 Confidentiality. The main guidelines have been covered elsewhere but it must be stressed that the contents of the records are of a highly confidential nature and even apparently innocuous information such as age, marital status and dates of attendance at the surgery must be treated with the same level of care as more obviously medical matters. Notes, records and reports should never be left where they can be seen inadvertently by unauthorised people. Conversations about reports and records must not take place where they can be overheard and information must never be given to people not entitled to receive it unless the patient has sanctioned the disclosure. This rule applies to everyone in the surgery who handles the records. In some surgeries records are locked in the filing system when the surgery is not in use.

4 Identification data. The receptionist rarely has to enter things in the notes herself. There are some occasions when staff make entries on drug sheets, but in the main it is the identification section of the medical

record that is the primary concern of the receptionist. This will contain the name, address, marital status, date of birth and National Health Service number, the first three of these can change from time to time. It is important that they are kept up to date and accurate or the doctor may get the wrong records, visit the wrong house, or write to the wrong address about an important health matter. Patients frequently tell receptionists about a change of address or marriage, and at such times there are other documents that might need altering. This may necessitate alterations to several documents; for other members of the family, age/sex record cards or other registers or computer listings.

In your practice, how do you handle records when patients attend the surgery or telephone?

What filing systems have you found most useful?

What kind of difficulties have you faced involving matters of confidentiality with reports and records?

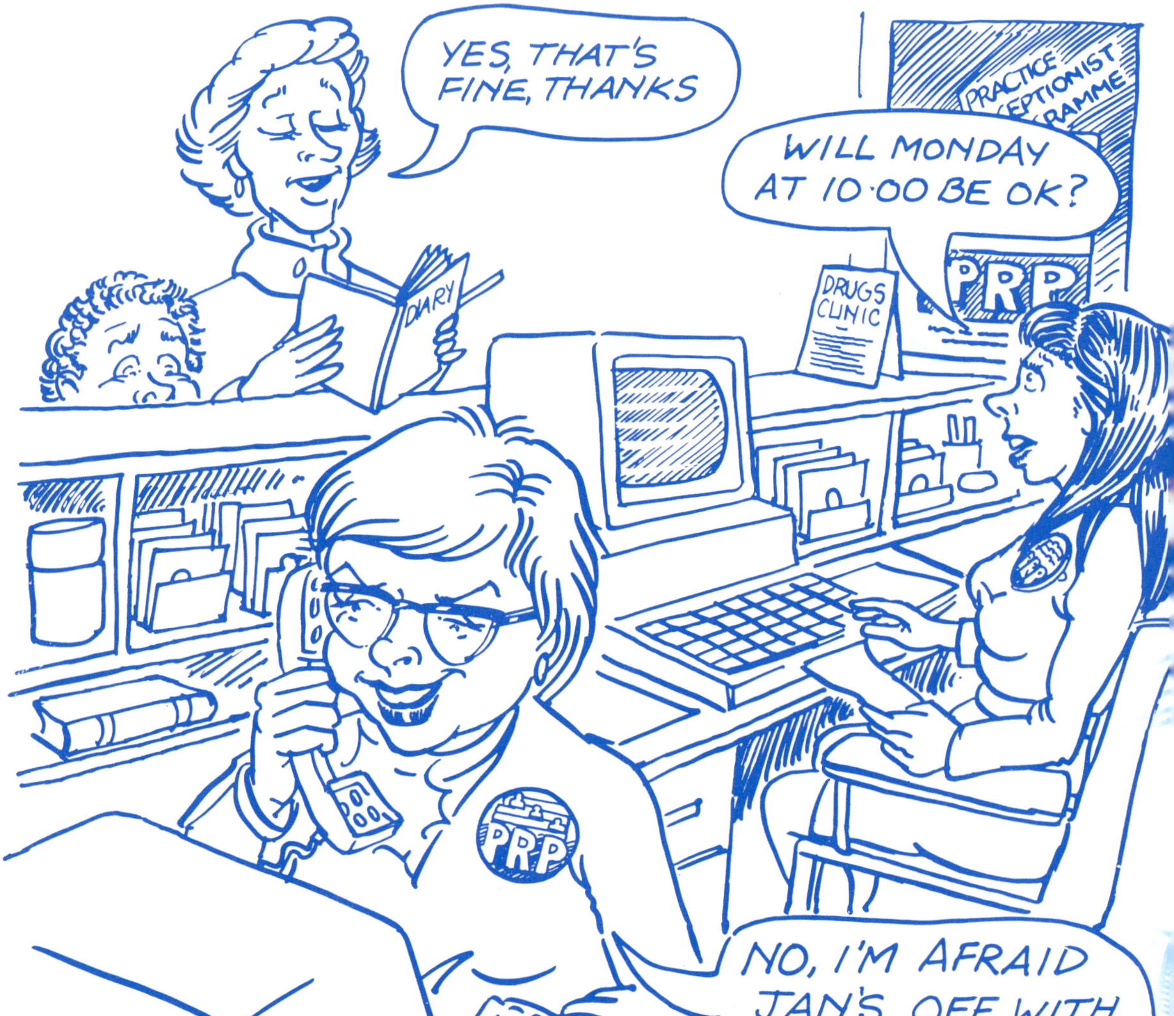
YES, THAT'S FINE, THANKS
WILL MONDAY AT 10·00 BE OK?
NO, I'M AFRAID JAN'S OFF WITH A SLIPPED DISK.
DIARY
DRUGS CLINIC
PRP

11 THE COMPUTER

During the next three or four years many practices will install a computer. At the same time most of the other institutions that we deal with – hospitals, laboratories, Family Practitioner Committees etc. – will be 'computerised' to some extent. So it is now important that the receptionist understands something about computers and what they can and cannot do.

WHAT CAN THE COMPUTER DO?

For most people it is sufficient to know what the computer can do and to use it for some specific tasks. Users may want to know how to correct simple faults but will not want to know much about what goes on inside. In this respect it is a bit like a car: the driver will want to use it and know how to change a tyre but will not want to know the details of the carburettor. In the practice the common tasks which are now being computerised include:

Maintaining the age/sex register
Running call and recall lists for categories of patients
Producing repeat prescriptions
Maintaining a disease register
Dealing with P.A.Y.E. of staff
Producing name and address stickers
Word processing

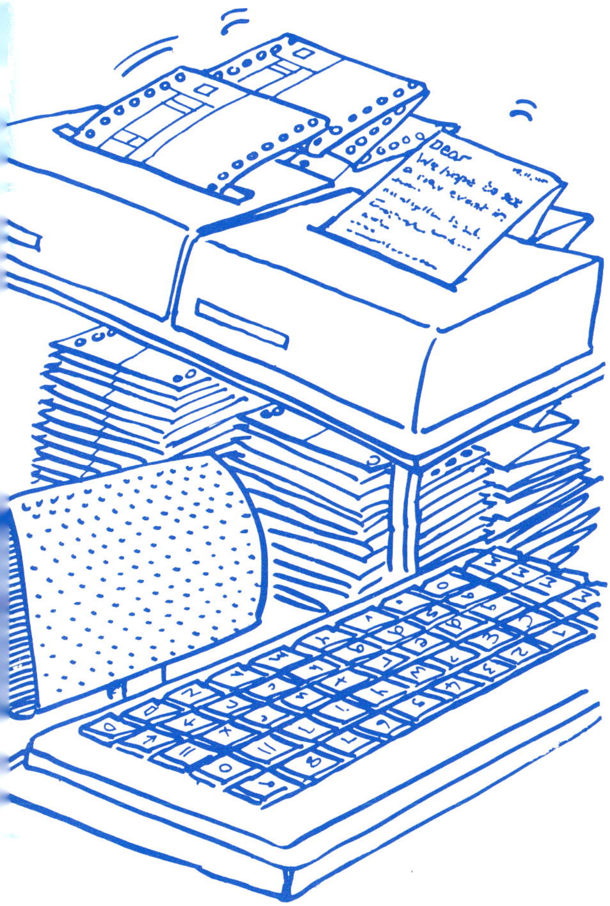

CONFIDENTIALITY

There has been a lot of anxiety expressed about the confidentiality of information stored on computers. It is not helped by stories in which small boys have gained access to the secrets of the Kremlin or the Pentagon. The computer in the surgery is more confidential than the ordinary written paper, but since computers can talk to each other the possibility of leaks occur. A partial protection against this is provided by the Data Protection Act. Broadly speaking the requirements of this apply to everyone who stores personal data about other people on a computer. If they do they must register under the Act and must take steps to see that the data is kept confidential, and that no unauthorised person can gain access to the information. In order to prevent incorrect or even libellous information being stored on computer there is a requirement of the Act that anyone may have unrestricted access to computer information about themselves, and can gain financial compensation if they are damaged by it. The computer does have some disadvantages. Although a very great deal of data may be stored on disks it is possible for it to be wiped off by accidents such as a power cut. This could be disastrous, so most users have a system of storing material on a back-up disk or tape which will be kept outside the machine. This should be done daily and very systematically and the most recent back-up should be kept outside the premises so that it is not lost in the event of a fire. In spite of these problems, the arrival of the computer on the medical scene is likely to make a huge contribution to standards of medical care by helping us to manage practices more efficiently.

COMPUTER HARDWARE

Computer hardware has been described as any part of a computer system that you can touch! As such it can be split into four functionally different units:

1. Input unit
2. Output unit
3. Storage unit
4. Central processing unit

1 The keyboard is the most commonly used method of input into a computer system, and is usually used in conjunction with a screen or VDU.

The style of the keyboard in most cases will conform with the standard QWERTY format found on typewriters (look at the first six letter keys at the top left-hand side of the keyboard).

2 To make the most of any computer system, any data or information processed by the computer must be accessible to the operator. More often than not this requires some kind of printer to be linked to the computer system.

Dot Matrix Printers

This is the most common method of printing particularly on the smaller mini and micro systems. It works by striking a Dot Matrix printhead against a ribbon to produce a character on a sheet of paper.

Daisy Wheel Printers

Daisy wheel printers operate at speeds of 16–80 cps and dominate the quality printing sector of the market. They offer good quality in a variety of typestyles and anything produced on them looks as though it could have been typed on an ordinary typewriter. Fully formed characters are located on the ends of spokes protruding from a central wheel, with the appearance of a large-faced flower, the spokes being like the petals on a daisy. Daisy wheels can be made of plastic (cheap but fragile) or metal (expensive and noisy, but longer lasting) and can be changed easily to give different typefaces.

3 When the computer is switched off the working memory is wiped clean and all data and programs are lost. So some form of permanent memory is required. The information held must be quickly accessible otherwise the advantages of fast processing can be lost. There are three main types of storage:

Solid-state memory based on silicon or garnet chips and resident in the computer.

Disk-based memory in which various technologies are used to transfer information to and from disk systems that may be integral with the computer or in connected disk drives.

Tape-based memory varying from simple audio cassettes to sophisticated mass data storage devices.

4 A computer is an electronic device, operating under the control of instructions stored in its own memory unit, which can accept and store information, perform arithmetic and logical operations on that information without human intervention, and produce output from the processing. This capacity to manipulate information with great speed and accuracy and to present it in many ways is possible because of the operations of the Central Processing Unit (C.P.U.). The C.P.U. is the heart of any computer system and can be subdivided into three functional units.

Control Unit

The control unit maintains order and controls activity in the C.P.U. It does not process or store data. It directs operations, interprets the instructions of a program in the computer's memory and produces signals that act as commands to circuits to execute the instructions. Other functions of the control unit are to communicate with an input device, e.g. a keyboard and the auxiliary backing store in order to begin the transfer of instructions and data into longer term memory and similarly to initiate the transfer of results from memory to an output device, e.g. a printer or the auxiliary backing store.

Arithmetic Logic Unit (ALU)

This part of the C.P.U. performs arithmetic computations and logical operations. The A.L.U. does not store data; it merely performs the necessary manipulations to achieve the results the user wants.

Main Memory

The main memory of the C.P.U. holds all instructions and data necessary for processing. It also holds intermediate and final results during manipulation. The program and the data to be used in it are transferred from an input device and/or auxiliary backing store to the main memory where it is stored until needed for processing. Data that is being processed and intermediate results of A.L.U. calculations are also held in this primary storage. After all computations and manipulations have been completed the final results remain in the memory. The control unit then directs them to be transferred to an output device or the auxiliary backing store (e.g. updating a file).

COMPUTER SOFTWARE

Computer software is the generic name for all the instructions that bring the hardware to life. These instructions are assembled into useful routines known as programs. Programs may be already 'in' the hardware or can be bought separately.

Software 'in' the machine is usually concerned with the control of the hardware and is called 'systems software', whereas software to perform specific functions, such as accounting or word processing is usually bought separately and called 'application software'.

Systems software

When a problem is to be solved with the aid of a computer certain procedures must be followed. Step by step instructions providing the problem solution are required. This series of instructions is known as a program. Systems programs co-ordinate the operations of all the computer circuitry. The operating system is a collection of programs designed to permit a computer system to manage its own operations. In many ways the operating system is the most important element of the system and its integrity and quality determine the effectiveness and efficiency of the computer.

Applications software

Many business tasks and problems are common to all firms and organisations. Typical examples are payroll, personnel, ledger transfers, credit control etc. Computer manufacturers realising that there will be a recurring market for such applications, will have available off the shelf packages (programs) to solve these problems.

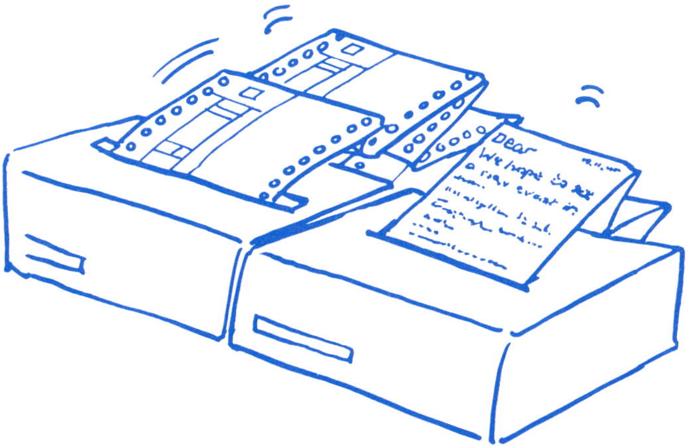

Acknowledgement The sections on Computer Hardware and Computer Software have been based on the Royal College of General Practitioners' course notes on Computer Appreciation.

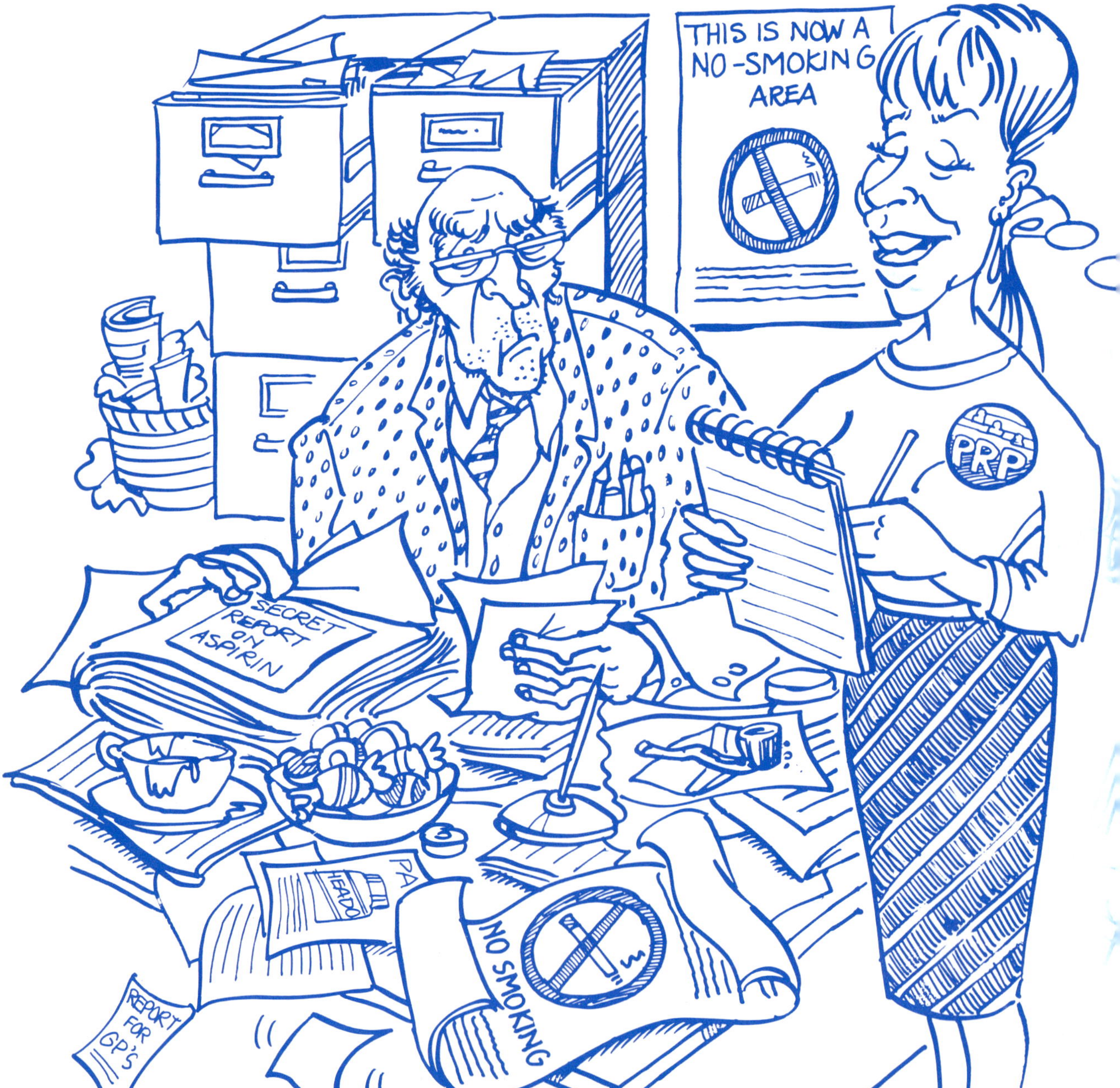
THIS IS NOW A NO-SMOKING AREA
SECRET REPORT ON ASPIRIN
PRP
NO SMOKING
REPORT FOR GP'S

12 EFFECTING CHANGE

Having undertaken the course and read the book this far you may now have lots of new ideas which you wish to apply. Your next hurdle is how to introduce your ideas so that they are accepted and put into practice.

Few of us work in practices where introduction of change 'from the ranks' is readily accepted. The very word 'change' is enough to set the teeth of some of our colleagues on edge, so we generally need to think carefully about how to go about the delicate task of introducing new ideas.

Perhaps the best way to analyse this problem is to take a piece of paper and list the ideas you have, grouping them into:

1. Changes which you can make to your own attitudes and methods of working which do NOT overlap with anyone else
2. Changes affecting yourself and your colleagues
3. Changes which will require the authorisation of partners/practice manager/senior receptionist

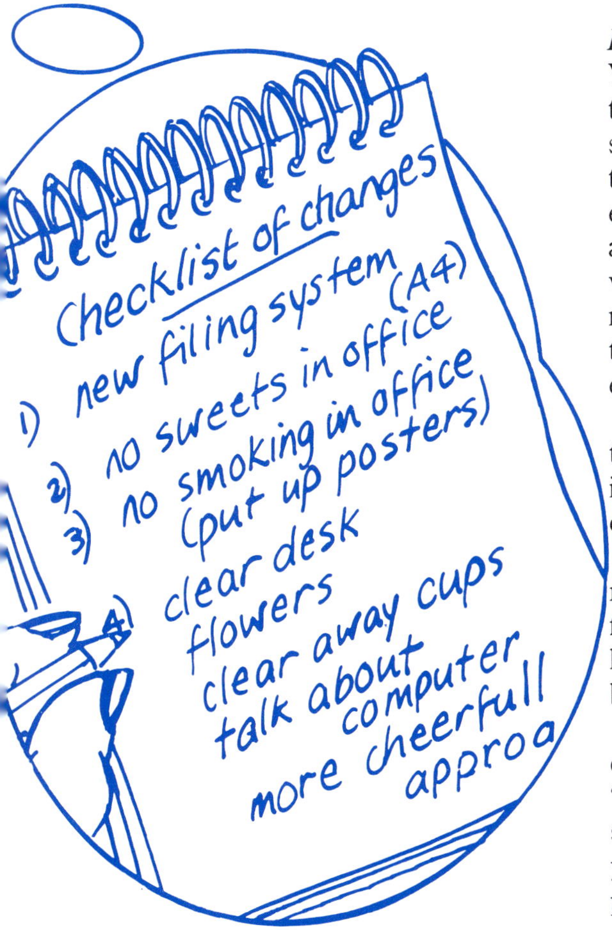

For example:

You may have taken to heart the fact that your tone of voice will be gentler and warmer if you smile as you speak. It will make no difference to your colleagues if you smile at the phone every time you answer it! But if your method of answering the phone is to face out into the waiting area, you may need to develop the new smiling habit by turning to one side, so that no-one can see you, and you do not feel embarrassed.

You do not need to tell anyone you intend to make this change to your own way of working, and you can go ahead with this sort of change as soon as you wish.

However, the second and third groups require careful handling if you do not wish to find yourself snubbed, causing reactions you had not expected, or getting remarks about not being able to leave anything as it is!

You will have learnt about how to handle difficult patients, and may have discussed 'bettering relationships' in the Teamwork session. This is where you draw together what you learned in those sessions and begin to practise the skills you have learned.

Several simple steps can help.

1 Think through the total effect of your idea. List the advantages, and disadvantages. List the people who must be advised of any changes, but who are not really part of the decision making process, eg health visitors, midwives, cleaners.

2 Assess the receptivity of those who will be most affected by the change you wish to introduce. Identify one person who you think will 'back you up' who is involved in the decision making processes of your practice (preferably the senior receptionist or practice manager, or the partner who shows most concern about how things are run in your department).

3 Mentally put yourself into the position of the person who is least receptive and try to see what their objections might be.

4 Think how you can 'put across' your idea. Prepare a simple outline, stating what the problem is, how you believe it can be overcome and the advantages and disadvantages of your suggestion. Practise sketching out any diagram that will help in your explanation of the principle or the detail, e.g. if you wish to revise the columns in the message book you might roughly head up a sheet of paper marking in the change you are suggesting as you explain. Do NOT make a really tidy diagram for your first approach. It will look as though you are trying too hard!

5 Suitable introductions might be:
'I've had an idea, what do you think of this?'
'What do you think of this suggestion?'
'Do you think it would be easier/simpler if we were to . . . . ?'
'I have noticed that we get into difficulties over . . . , would it help if we were to . . . . . ?'
Try to find ways of phrasing your ideas, using open ended questions such as 'What?', 'Where?', 'When?', 'How?', 'Who?' and couched in such a way that others hear that you are making a suggestion, not producing a 'fait accompli' or stating 'This is how it WILL be done'.

6 Choose someone whom you trust and discuss your idea with them confidentially. Listen to their comments on your idea and modify your method and presentation if necessary.

7 CHOOSE YOUR TIME FOR SAYING SOMETHING VERY CAREFULLY. This applies equally to colleagues and employers. The end of a busy morning when everyone is tired is not the time for introducing bright new ideas, nor is nine o'clock in the morning – if you work in the average surgery! So don't go racing in fresh from the previous evening's session and expect anyone to be really open to listening to you. Once you have been interrupted in your flow it will be more difficult to regain attention.

Similarly, when approaching a doctor, wait for an appropriate opportunity. It may even be necessary to ask when you might have five minutes of his time. When the inevitable 'What about?' comes, be prepared to say something to the effect that you have an idea you would like him to consider, but you wish to have time to explain it fully. Resist the temptation to be drawn at that point. If it is the first time you have made such a move, speak to the doctor when he is on his own — you are less likely to get 'wise-guy' cracks which would embarrass you in front of your colleagues.

If you have Staff or Practice Meetings this may be the best opportunity to introduce ideas, particularly if you work in a team where there are many part-timers, you will avoid someone telling you they did not know there had been any change in the system.

8 Therefore, when you are successful, don't forget to ensure that EVERYONE knows about the change. There is nothing worse than a success which is then slapped in the face because someone did not know about it, and bad feeling generated as a result can raise further obstacles to future developments. If you have a practice procedure file, update the relevant pages. Otherwise, in the event of the change being somewhat complex, write out a memo and circulate to all concerned, so that any misunderstanding can be discussed.

9 DON'T GIVE UP if your first attempt falls flat. Analyse why and chalk up the attempt to experience. Then try again.

Be extremely sensitive towards the feelings of everyone. Don't be afraid to get doctor support, or even to ask the doctor to put forward an idea as his if that is going to oil the wheels.

Start with something small. Preferably something which will make life easier without involving anyone else in extra work! If you build up a little set of improvements, your confidence will grow and experience will tell you how best to tackle various situations. Be prepared to discuss other ideas that may surface as a result of your suggestion, and compromise gracefully if appropriate. Don't be put off by a negative response and unco-operative attitudes. Think it through and try again later with an amended proposal if you are confident you are on the right track. Remember — there is no forward movement without turbulence.

Ideally we hope to bring about change smoothly. It is possible to have a team where change does not cause fear and distress. But most of us work in an environment where any change, no matter how small, is seen to be a threat by someone. Therefore, if we wish to progress we must be aware of the feelings of those with whom we work, allow for this, and work around it. Often we may put forward an idea which is apparently rejected, only to re-surface two years later from someone else. When this happens you will know that, even if it was only subconsciously, you were being listened to. We need as much skill and patience to introduce change as to deal with the most difficult patient, yet at a totally different pitch and level.

Finally, a sting in the tail! Are *you* really open to change? Change begins with you. You must also be prepared to change your ways, habits and attitudes. If you are busy trying to get other people to do what *you* will not do, *everyone* is going to get frustrated!

We must be aware that the objective of change is to improve situations. If a problem were easy to solve it would have been solved long ago. Whatever difficulties you face (many of them are long-established) you will need to tackle them bit by bit, rather than 'head on'. You need practice, optimism, realism and courage to face facts, plan our strategy, and start the wheels in motion. There will be setbacks, stumbling blocks and discouragement. But there will also be successes, which will encourage us and give us a sense of job satisfaction. You will be happier doing your work as you see your working environment providing the most caring and effective service you can give.

Index